tur

7

0

Between Cultures

Asians are an integral part of Western society and Britain itself is now permanently a multi-racial and multi-cultural society. Almost all young Asians have been born and/or brought up in Britain and can no longer be considered to be 'immigrants', 'foreigners' or 'outsiders'. Using empirical data, *Between Cultures* examines the position of young Asians in education, employment and other fields as well as the attitudes and behaviour of young Asians and Asian parents in relation to education, religion, the family and marriage, and other cultural issues. It also considers the responses of policy makers, professionals and the Asian communities to the needs of young Asians and looks at the participation of young Asians in the political process. Contextualising the material, it compares the situation of young Asians with that of young whites from the same geographical areas.

Between Cultures presents a unique and comprehensive analysis of the changing situation of young Asians over the last twenty years. It will appeal to students of anthropology, sociology and social policy.

Muhammad Anwar is Research Professor in the Centre for Research in Ethnic Relations (CRER), University of Warwick, having formerly been Director of CRER (1989–94) and Head of Research, Commission for Racial Equality (1981–9).

Between Cultures

Continuity and Change in the Lives of Young Asians

Muhammad Anwar

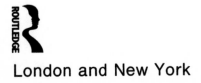

London and New York

First published 1998 by Routledge
11 New Fetter Lane, London EC4P 4EE

Simultaneously published in the USA and Canada
by Routledge
29 West 35th Street, New York, NY 10001

© 1998 Muhammad Anwar

Typeset in Times by Pure Tech India Ltd, Pondicherry
Printed and bound in Great Britain by Creative Print and
Design (Wales), Ebbw Vale

British Library Cataloguing in Publication Data

A catalogue record for this book is available from the British Library

Library of Congress Cataloging in Publication Data
Anwar, Muhammad, 1945–
    Between cultures: continuity and change in the lives of young
Asians / Muhammad Anwar.
        p.   cm.
    Includes bibliographical references and index.
    1. Asians–Great Britain–Social life and customs. 2. Great
Britain–Race relations. I. Title.
DA125.A84A58   1998
305.895'041–dc21   97–18727
                                                            CIP

ISBN 0–415–04647–5 (hbk)
ISBN 0–415–04648–3 (pbk)

To my father
and in memory of my mother

Contents

Tables

Preface

Britain is now permanently a multi-racial and multi-cultural society. Asians are an integral part of British society. In this book, the position of young Asians in education, employment and other fields is examined. The book also includes an analysis of the attitudes and behaviour of young Asians and their parents to education, religion and other cultural issues by using empirical data. It is the first comprehensive book to analyse the changing situation of young Asians over the last twenty years.

The origins of this book go back to 1975 when I undertook a national study of relationships between generations in the Asian communities in Britain. This was published as *Between Two Cultures* (1976) by the then Community Relations Commission. As a follow-up to this work, the Commission for Racial Equality decided to undertake a comparative study of young people, including whites. I designed and supervised this study in 1983 and 1984. It also included a sample of Asian young people and Asian parents, and additional questions were asked about religio-cultural aspects in order to make the survey findings comparable to the 1975 survey (for details see Appendix). More recently, I carried out, in the early 1990s, some ethnographic research in Birmingham and other areas which were included in the 1975 and 1983/4 surveys. Information on some of these relevant issues has also recently become available from the Policy Studies Institute's (PSI's) Fourth Survey of Ethnic Minorities (Modood *et al.* 1997), for which I was a member of the Advisory Group. All these surveys and other sources of information, including the 1991 Census, are used in the book.

In the preparation of this book many individuals and organisations have helped me and it is impossible to mention all their names. I am grateful to all these. I would like to acknowledge the help I received from my colleagues when I was Head of Research at the Commission for Racial Equality, until my move to the University of Warwick in 1989 as Director of the Centre for Research in Ethnic Relations (CRER). I would like to thank my colleagues at CRER for their help during my work on this book, in particular David Owen, Zig Layton-Henry, Beryl Pine-Coffin and Tahir Abbas.

I would also like to thank Gurbakhsh Hundal for preparing the manuscript, and Rose Goodwin, Claudette Brennan and Caroline Oakman for their help.

I must thank Heather Gibson of Routledge for encouraging me to write this book.

Finally, I am grateful to my wife, Saeeda, and daughters, Fatima and Aisha, for their support and patience during the writing of this book.

Muhammad Anwar
University of Warwick

Terminology

1 The terms 'Asian' and 'South Asian' are used interchangeably throughout the book, and refer to people whose origin is mainly from the Indian subcontinent, including East African Asians.

2 The term 'coloured' was commonly used in the early period of post-1945 migration, in official documents and also by some researchers. I prefer to use 'non-white' and 'ethnic minorities' for people whose origin is mainly from the New Commonwealth except where official and other sources are quoted with the original terms.

ABOUT THE TABLES

1 Percentages are rounded to the nearest whole number and therefore some tables do not add up to 100. Other tables do not add up to 100 because a few respondents did not give a clear answer.

2 A dash (—) is used for zero per cent. Less than 1.00 per cent is shown as an asterisk (*).

3 All Census information is Crown Copyright.

Chapter 1

Introduction

Migration to Britain is not a new phenomenon. For a long time, the country has received and absorbed a large number of people from other countries while many Britons have gone abroad to colonies as rulers, administrators, soldiers, businessmen and missionaries. Those who came to Britain in early and more recent periods were mainly white people and included: Germans, Dutch, Flemings, Walloons, Huguenots, Irish, Jews and Poles. For example, in 1851, there were 727,326 Irish immigrants in Britain, making up 2.9 per cent of the population of England and Wales and 7.2 per cent of the population of Scotland (Jackson 1963). Between 1875 and 1914, it is estimated that 120,000 Jews came to Britain from Eastern Europe, particularly Russia, to escape persecution there. These immigrants were largely poor and unskilled and the majority of them settled in the East End of London.

After World War II, about 460,000 foreigners entered Britain. They included 115,000 Poles who came under the Polish Resettlement Scheme. In addition to a number of former prisoners of war, Germans, Ukrainians and Italians who entered Britain, the British government recruited 90,000 European Voluntary Workers (EVWs), mostly from refugee camps in Germany. The EVWs and other immigrants after the war met with considerable hostility from British labour (see p. 9). However, over a period, all these workers, who were white, were slowly absorbed into the labour market and more workers were needed in some sectors of the industry. This gap was filled by workers from the New Commonwealth. Due to their colonial links and, in particular, their participation in World War II, some of the several thousand soldiers and seamen from the West Indies and India decided to stay in Britain, and others came back to work after the war, since under the Commonwealth rules they had free entry into Britain. They were initially welcomed by the British people as allies who had defended their national survival (Cabinet Papers 1950). The process of mass migration of non-white workers started slowly, but, during the 1950s, the number of immigrants from the West Indies increased, reaching an annual rate of 30,000 in 1955 and 1956, when some concern was expressed about the number of 'coloured' immigrants (Anwar 1995). As the pressure for, and debate on, immigration control grew, more and more West Indians migrated to Britain to beat the impending ban. For example, between the beginning of 1961 and the middle of 1962, when the Commonwealth Immigrants Act came into force, 98,000 persons entered Britain from the West Indies. The immigration of workers from India and Pakistan started later than that from the West Indies, but also reached a very high level from 1960 onwards, as people tried to enter Britain while there was still time. As a result, the number of New Commonwealth immigrants more than doubled in the inter-censal period of 1951–61, from 256,000 to 541,000.

In 1955, just under 8,000 people from India and Pakistan entered Britain, while this number rose to 49,000 in 1961 and 44,000 for the first six months of 1962 up to the introduction of the Act. As a result of this pattern of migration from the Indian subcontinent, the number of Indians and Pakistanis increased substantially in the inter-censal period of 1951–61 from 36,000 to 106,000. Those who entered Britain before the 1962 Act were predominantly economically active persons and the overwhelming majority of them were men.

In the beginning, the migration was unorganised, but, later on, it resulted in chain migration where friends and relatives were encouraged and helped by pioneer migrants to follow them (Anwar 1979). Chain migration can be defined as the movement in which prospective migrants learn of opportunities, are provided with transportation and have initial accommodation and employment arranged by means of primary social relationships with previous migrants (MacDonald and MacDonald 1962). It was exemplified in the various forms of sponsorship and patronage of friends and relatives by those Asians who were already in Britain. This resulted in mass migration of people from the Indian subcontinent. Mass migration in turn resulted in the establishment of institutions, agents and organisations to facilitate the migration. In this way, even after the 1962 Act, the introduction of the voucher system reinforced the sponsorship and patronage of friends and relatives because the migrants already in Britain were in a position to obtain vouchers for their kin and friends. Later immigration legislation and debates on immigration from the Commonwealth forced the migrants to bring their dependents to Britain because of the fear of losing their right to entry.

It is worth mentioning here that, in addition to voluntary movement of people, some institutional arrangements helped the process of migration too. For example, in India and Pakistan, British textile and other companies advertised for workers and some workers were directly recruited. This also resulted in chain migration of Indians, Pakistanis and later on Bangladeshis from the same areas. The Pakistanis who work in Lancashire and Yorkshire textile mills and the Indians in the car industry and foundries in the West Midlands have been part of such a migration process. Two other factors which contributed to the migration of Indians and Pakistanis to Britain were the partition of British India in 1947, when Pakistan was created, and the construction of the Mangla Dam in Pakistan. In both cases large numbers of people were displaced and some of them looked for economic opportunities in Britain and other countries.

At the time of the partition in 1947, a large-scale movement of population took place between India and Pakistan. Under an agreement, almost all of the Muslim, Hindu and Sikh populations of East and West Punjab were exchanged and there was also a large exchange of Muslim and Hindu population between East (now Bangladesh) and West Bengal. Many Muslims from all over India, especially from its northern parts, took refuge in Pakistan and similarly Hindus and Sikhs were settled in India. Surveys have shown that many of these displaced people came to Britain (Anwar 1979). This migration fits into Petersen's (1958) category of the impelled-flight type. More recent examples of such forced migration include what has happened in Bosnia, Croatia and Serbia, where ethnic cleansing took place in the mid-1990s.

The other group of displaced people was the Mirpuris. It is estimated that about 100,000 people were moved from the area in the early 1960s when the Mangla Dam was constructed. At the end of the 1950s and the beginning of the 1960s the villagers of the proposed dam area were given compensation. Some were given land in the Punjab, others received cash and settled in various areas of Pakistan. But some who had friends and relatives in

Britain used the compensation money to come to Britain to find work. Therefore, the presence of a large number of Mirpuris in Britain is a direct result of displacement by the dam and an arrangement at government level to admit them into Britain (Allen 1971). No doubt this was not the only factor, but my research shows that this certainly contributed to the large-scale migration of Mirpuris in conjunction with the voucher system introduced in the 1962 Act. The nature of the migration changed after the Act (Ballard 1996).

The voucher system gave the opportunity to those who were already in Britain to arrange jobs and vouchers for their relatives and friends, but dependents of those already settled in this country were allowed to come without vouchers. As a result the balance shifted between workers and dependents entering Britain. Between July 1962, when the new Act became operative, and December 1968 only 77,966 voucher holders were admitted, compared with 257,200 dependents, from the New Commonwealth countries (Deakin 1970). This means a drastic decline in the number of migrants coming as workers. My analysis shows that the net immigration from the West Indies, India and Pakistan between 1955 and 1968 was 669,690 (Anwar 1979). The number of people arriving for settlement from all the New Commonwealth countries between 1969 and 1977 was 318,521; of these, 259,646 came as dependents and only 58,875 were male workers, thus continuing the decline in the number of immigrants entering as workers (Anwar 1986). This pattern of decline applied also to dependents and has continued. In 1972, for example, the number of men accepted for settlement on arrival was 14,100 and in 1982 this was reduced to a trickle – 1,700. At the same time the number of dependent women and children was reduced from over 45,000 in 1972 to just over 15,000 in 1983. This downward trend between 1971 and 1983 is also clear from Table 1.1.

It is interesting to point out that in 1984 out of a total of 51,000 immigrants accepted for settlement, 24,800 – less than half – were from the New Commonwealth. In 1988 this number was reduced to 22,700. However, we know from empirical evidence that dependents of legally settled migrants face a lot of difficulties in getting entry to Britain (CRE 1985a, 1989a). On the other hand it is worth mentioning here that between 1971 and 1983 more people left Britain than entered it. Overall the net loss of migration during this period was almost half a million (465,000), mainly as a result of

Table 1.1 Immigration from the New Commonwealth, 1971–83: all acceptances for settlement (thousands)

Year	Total accepted for settlement	Men	Women	Children
1971	44.3	10.9	16.7	16.7
1972	68.5	17.4	23.8	26.9
1973	30.3	5.3	13.5	11.5
1974	42.5	14.5	17.3	10.7
1975	53.3	16.6	21.4	15.2
1976	55.1	16.1	22.1	16.4
1977	44.1	10.7	19.6	13.8
1978	42.9	11.8	18.6	12.5
1979	37.2	9.9	16.5	10.8
1980	33.7	8.9	14.4	10.4
1981	31.4	7.4	13.3	10.7
1982	30.4	7.3	13.2	9.9
1983	27.5	6.3	13.0	8.1

Source: Home Office 1984

emigration to Australia, New Zealand, the United States, Canada, South Africa and the EU countries.

In 1992, the overall acceptances for settlement from the New Commonwealth, including removal of conditions of those already settled in Britain, numbered 27,900 (52 per cent of all acceptances), from old Commonwealth countries 3,120 (6 per cent) and from other countries 21,760 (41 per cent) (Home Office 1993–6). The acceptances from the Indian subcontinent were 15,070. Out of these almost 10,000 were wives and children and only 3,350 husbands were accepted. In 1993, the number of people accepted for settlement from the Indian subcontinent came down to 14,120 (Home Office 1993–6). Once again the proportion of dependents is very high in this figure. Only 8 per cent of all immigrants were accepted for settlement on the basis of employment and in their own right. Between June 1995 and June 1996, out of a total number of acceptances for settlement of 57,660, only 24 per cent came from the Indian subcontinent and the pattern of migrant categories was similar to 1993, with a downward trend (Home Office 1993–6). This pattern of migration shows that the large-scale immigration of workers from the Indian subcontinent and other New Commonwealth countries has been over for a long time. Therefore, it is a myth that Britain is receiving large-scale non-white immigration.

However, the topic of non-white immigration to Britain still provokes unnecessary political and media reactions.

In addition to migration of Asians from the Indian subcontinent, a significant number of Asians have also migrated from East Africa, after the policy of Africanisation in many states in the region. Most of them were British passport holders and were also 'twice migrants' (Bhachu 1986). This migration mainly started in the 1970s when East African Asians were forced to leave African countries. For example, the president of Uganda, Idi Amin, expelled over 29,000 Asians who migrated to Britain in 1972. In 1971, the estimated number of Asians from East Africa resident in Britain was about 45,000. However, with more expulsions from African countries, the number of East African Asians in 1981 was estimated at about 180,000 (1971 and 1981 Censuses: see OPCS 1983). Because the 1991 Census included an ethnic question, it appears that most East African Asians identified themselves as either Indians or Pakistanis. Some may have identified themselves as 'other Asians'. Therefore, it is difficult to come up with a reasonable estimate of East African Asians in the late 1990s.

Unlike those Asians who came direct from the Indian subcontinent as single men, most East African Asians entered Britain as family units. The majority of them were also educated, spoke good English and had commercial, professional or business experience before entering Britain. In the case of Ugandan Asians in 1972, the Heath government set up the Uganda Resettlement Board (URB) to help with the exodus of a large number within a brief period. The refugees came as extended family units and were housed initially in sixteen transit camps to help their settlement. However, most of them eventually settled in areas of high Asian concentrations where, in some cases, they were helped by friends and relatives. This happened despite the opposition to the resettlement of refugees in particular areas (Bristow 1976; Dines 1973; Ward 1973; Kohler 1973) and the doubts of the electorate over the admission of refugees.

Another estimate showed that the East African Asian population in Britain was about 68,000 before the arrival of the Ugandan Asians (OPCS Immigrant Statistics Unit 1975). This included those who had migrated voluntarily and those who were forced to migrate because of Africanisation policies, particularly in Kenya, Uganda and Malawi. They were mainly concentrated in the East Midlands and Greater London regions. This concentration of East African Asians has not changed in the last two decades.

It is relevant to mention another small group of South Asians who migrated to Britain via the West Indies. They were taken to the West Indies as indentured labourers after the formal abolition of slavery. They are sometimes called Indo-Caribbeans and often seen as Asians by white people in Britain. The Indians from Trinidad and Guyana, the largest group, are estimated at between 22,800 and 30,400 (Boodhoo and Baksh 1981; Vertovec 1994). They are not concentrated in Britain except in some areas of South London and any movement by them has taken place within Greater London. It appears that, unlike those of other Asian migrants, the children of Indo-Caribbeans are almost exclusively British-born and raised (Vertovec 1994). This has implications for whether these people identify themselves as 'Asians' or British Indo-Caribbean. Most Asians do not have a functional contact with this group, except some young people who participate in general British Asian youth culture. However, there are other groups such as Indo-Mauritians and Indo-Fijians in London (Lingayah 1987) who are in a similar situation. The indications are that those groups of young people identify more with Britain than with the Indian subcontinent, while carrying on their cultural traditions with the help of their religio-cultural associations.

It is worth stressing here that, while the mass migration of Asians has taken place since 1945, their presence in Britain goes back to the seventeenth century (Fryer 1984; Visram 1986). The migration of Indians started in the early twentieth century among seamen (Aurora 1967; Desai 1963). It is estimated that in Birmingham the Indian population grew from 100 in 1939 to 1,000 in 1945, largely because of the movement of seamen into the city (Rose *et al.* 1969). It was also estimated that, in 1949, there were about 1,000 Indian doctors practising in Britain (Kondapi 1951). There were also Asian pedlars, mainly Sikhs, in Britain before 1945 and their origins go back to the time of World War I.

The estimated population of the main Asian groups between 1951 and 1981 is presented in Table 1.2. It shows that the population increase, in particular between 1961 and 1971, was very significant. As mentioned above this was the period when a substantial mass migration took place.

The 1951 to 1971 Censuses used the birthplace for estimates. The 1981 Census figures were calculated on the basis of the 'head of household's birthplace', which excluded Asians who were born in England and Wales and had set up their own households.

Table 1.2 South Asian estimated population in England and
Wales, 1951–81 (thousands)

Country of birth/ ethnic group	1951	1961	1971	1981
India	30,800	81,400	240,730	673,704
Pakistan*	5,000	24,900	127,565	295,461
Bangladeshi	—	—	—	64,562
East African Asians	—	—	45,000	181,321
Total	35,800	106,300	413,295	1,215,048

Sources: Rose et al. 1969; 1981 Census reports
* Figures for 1951–71 include Bangladeshis as East Pakistan was then part of Pakistan.

Therefore, the figure for the 1981 Census, though useful, was never accurate. The 1991 British Census for the first time included an ethnic question by using nine categories. As a result that Census provided the most comprehensive information, both national and local, regarding the demographic and socio-economic position of South Asian and other ethnic minority groups in Britain (Anwar 1990). The 1991 Census revealed that there were almost 1.5 million people of South Asian origin living in Britain (see Chapter 2). I estimate that the South Asian origin population in 1997 was just over 1.7 million.

However, before we look at the settlement patterns of South Asians, it would be useful to analyse political and public reactions to Asians and other non-white migration to Britain. This is important for the context in which we will look at the position of young Asians in the society and their attitudes to various issues.

POLITICAL AND PUBLIC REACTIONS TO MIGRATION

It is worth pointing out that, before the mass migration of non-whites, workers from Ireland and, after the Industrial Revolution, the Jews who migrated to Britain from Eastern Europe also faced hostility from the local population. Employers kept Irish and English workers separate to avoid conflict at work and there was frequent discrimination with regard to jobs and housing (Engels 1952). 'No Irish' signs were common in England. The majority of the Jews settled in the East End of London where they were exploited by employers and landlords. Fear of competition for jobs and housing led to hostility from the local population. Mass demonstrations against migration were organised and the new-comers were accused of causing society's ills. The campaign resulted in Britain's first restrictive legislation on immigration, the Aliens Act of 1905 and the Aliens Restriction Act of 1914. After World War II, between 1946 and 1951, the EVWs, Poles and other immigrants from Europe also met with considerable hostility from British workers. The opposition of British workers to the employ-ment of foreigners was strong enough to bring about the latter's complete exclusion from some work situations. This was despite the preference for finding (possibly European) workers to meet shortages, as recommended by the Royal Commission on Popula-tion which reported in 1949 (Royal Commission on Population 1949). The Commission argued that immigrant workers with the same religion and race could be welcomed without reserve, imply-ing that non-white workers would create problems. This notion was also supported by a Political and Economic Planning (PEP) report on population policy at the time, which argued that it would be extremely difficult for non-white immigrants to be absorbed into society (PEP 1948). This clearly applied to South Asian immigrants on both counts, namely race and religion.

As a result of these reports in 1948 and 1949, and after the arrival of the *Empire Windrush*, the SS *Orbita* and the SS *Georgia* with Afro-Caribbean immigrants on board in 1948, there was some interest in the House of Commons, in the form of some MPs questioning relevant ministers on immigration. As a result of this interest the government set up an inter-departmental working party to look into the possibilities of employing in Britain the surplus personnel of certain colonial territories. This working party and another inter-departmental committee in 1950 recommended ways and means of keeping colonial immigrants out of Britain. The Labour government of the time, in its cabinet meetings, discussed the immigration of non-whites in May and June 1950. It concluded that no decision should be taken, following the advice of the Home Secretary that the numbers were small and that the legislation to control immigration could be controversial (Cabinet Papers 1950). Between 1951 and 1955 the immigration issue was raised by some MPs (*Hansard* 1951–5) and a few discussions took place in Cabinet meetings. It was in November 1955 that a Committee of Ministers was appointed to consider what form legislation should take, 'if it were to be decided that legislation to control the entry into the

United Kingdom of British subjects from overseas should be introduced ... how any such control would be justified to Parliament and to the public, and to the Commonwealth countries concerned, (Cabinet Papers 1956). No action was taken as a result but the Committee felt that non-white immigration was a problem and that it should be kept under review.

By the late 1950s there was some reaction to non-white immigrants in local areas and there was discrimination in employment and housing in particular. However, those incidents did not appear on the national public or political agenda except in the discussions mentioned above. The turning point was the race riots in Nottingham and Notting Hill in London in August and September 1958, which made headlines in the national newspapers and the broadcasting media, and then the issue of immigration control was discussed widely. A Gallup poll, taken immediately after the riots, found that 92 per cent of the respondents had read about them, 27 per cent blamed blacks, the largest number (35 per cent) blamed both whites and blacks, and, as a result, a great majority of the respondents favoured immigration control, with a minority opposing it. The Labour Party condemned the riots, issued a statement opposing racial discrimination, and was also against immigration control. On the other hand, the Conservative Party, which had opposed control in the past, responded to public pressure and, after the 1959 general election, introduced a bill to control Commonwealth immigration. This became law on 1 July 1962 and broke the tradition of free entry to the UK of Commonwealth and colonial subjects. Since then, the issue of immigration of non-whites and now ethnic minorities has often been in the political and public domain, one way or the other.

After the 1962 Act was passed, the 1964 general election provided an opportunity for the Conservative Party to proclaim the benefits of the Act and for Labour to accuse the Conservatives of using immigration as an excuse for their poor performance in education and housing (Foot 1965). However, in Smethwick, in the West Midlands, Patrick Gordon-Walker, Labour Shadow Foreign Secretary, was defeated by Peter Griffiths of the Conservative Party, who ran an anti-immigration campaign (Hartley-Brewer 1965). It appeared that, in some other areas, anti-immigration candidates had also attracted support. Griffiths was never repudiated by the Conservative Party leadership and in fact, after losing his Smethwick seat at the 1966 general election, when Labour returned with an increased majority, he returned to Parliament in 1979 as the member for Portsmouth North (Layton-Henry 1992). This is when the Conservative Party won the election under Margaret Thatcher, who had also spoken against the immigration of non-whites in 1978 (see p. 12).

The Labour government had passed the first Race Relations Act in 1965, which established the Race Relations Board (RRB). This co-ordinated the work of nine regional conciliation committees, which were established to deal with complaints of racial discrimination in places of public resort. However, the majority of the complaints received were about employment, housing and the police, and these were outside the scope of the Act. As a result of more evidence of discrimination, the Labour government passed the Race Relations Act of 1968 to tackle racial discrimination in employment, housing and the provision of goods, facilities and services, including education (Anwar 1991b). This Act set up the Community Relations Commission (CRC) in addition to the RRB. However, on the other hand, the Labour government also passed the Commonwealth Immigration Act in 1968, restricting the entry of mainly East African Asians with British nationality. The Act, which was passed within a week, distinguished between British citizens who were 'patrials' and those who were not, and applied the voucher system to British citizens who were 'non-patrials', thus creating a two-tier British citizenship. In some quarters, particularly among Asians, this was seen as an act of betrayal. But it appears that the Labour Party was ignoring its principles and was responding to some sections of the public on the immigration issue.

In this context, it must be mentioned that Enoch Powell, MP for Wolverhampton South West, kept writing in newspapers and making speeches against large-scale non-white immigration in 1967, and then made his 'rivers of blood' speech on 20 April 1968 (Cosgrave 1990). Edward Heath, the Conservative Party leader at the time, declared Powell's speech to be racialist in tone and dropped him from his Shadow Cabinet. However, this did not stop Powell getting some public support and making non-white immigrants and their British-born children a topic for his speeches for a long time. Heath's government, elected at the 1970 general election, passed the Immigration Act in 1971, following the Conservative Party manifesto. This Act extended the 1962 and 1968 immigration legislation and made the entry of non-whites to Britain even more difficult. Then came the expulsion of Ugandan Asians by President Idi Amin in September and October 1972, as mentioned above. There was intense media coverage of this development and Powell and his supporters used the opportunity to exploit public feelings regarding non-white immigrants. As a consequence, the right-wing Monday Club started the 'Halt Immigration Now' campaign in 1972.

The issue of non-white immigration also led to the formation of several other active anti-immigrant organisations. The first two to oppose immigration were in Birmingham and Southall, formed in 1960: the Birmingham Immigration Control Association and the Southall Residents Association. The National Front was founded in 1966 and started contesting elections particularly in the 1970s on an anti-immigrant platform. Several books and articles have been written on the National Front (Taylor 1982; Walker 1977; Anwar 1986), and here it is worth mentioning that it received some electoral support for a period from right-wing supporters of other political parties and certainly received a lot of publicity in the media. For example, its candidate Martin Webster saved his deposit in the West Bromwich parliamentary by-election in May 1973. However, later on, the National Front was totally rejected by the British public at the ballot box, which gives the best criterion for estimating support (Anwar 1994). For example, in the October 1974 general election, with 90 candidates, the National Front's average vote received was 3.1 per cent; in 1979 with 303 candidates it received 1.4 per cent; in 1983 with 60 candidates it received 1 per cent; and in 1992 with 14 candidates its average vote was only 0.9 per cent per candidate. Another anti-immigrant organisation was the British Campaign to Stop Immigration (BCSI), which contested the 1972 Parliamentary by-election in Rochdale (Anwar 1973) followed by local elections in Rochdale and Bradford (Anwar 1974, 1975). This organisation did not last for a long time but it certainly created bad feelings against and problems for Asians in some areas of Yorkshire and Lancashire.

During the 1970s, the Conservative Party received many resolutions on immigration for its annual conferences. As a result of 140 resolutions on immigration at the Party conference in 1976, the Conservative Shadow Home Secretary, William Whitelaw, declared that the party would work towards ending the post-war immigration. This was followed by Margaret Thatcher in an interview on the television programme *World in Action*. In this she said that people were really afraid that Britain might be swamped by people of different cultures: 'we do have to hold out the prospect of an end to immigration except, of course, for compassionate cases' (Granada Television 30 January 1978). This interview received wide coverage in the media and some of the articles were very critical of Margaret Thatcher's remarks. However, it brought the issue of Asian and other non-white people in Britain on to the national public and political agenda.

Several events in the 1980s and 1990s, helped to bring about a focus on non-white people and on immigration, including inner-city riots in Bristol in 1980, in Brixton and Toxteth in 1981 (Anwar 1981; Scarman 1981), and in Handsworth and Tottenham in 1985; the issue of Hong Kong British passport holders and other British Dependent Territories when the Nationality Act 1981 was going through Parliament; the British Nationality (Hong Kong) Bill in 1990, during which Norman Tebbit MP (now Lord Tebbit) proposed a 'cricket test' of the loyalty of ethnic minorities in Britain; the Rushdie affair in 1989; and the more recent issue of refugees and asylum-seekers from former Yugoslavia and other troubled regions in the world. All these events received extensive coverage in the media, and the tone was generally negative and anti-foreigner.

In September 1993 the first ever victory of the British National Party (BNP) in a local council by-election, in Millwall in Tower Hamlets, which has a high Bangladeshi Asian population, also received wide media coverage. The event highlighted racist attitudes and behaviour in the area. One ICM opinion poll for the *Sunday Express* found that more than 80 per cent of those questioned were concerned about immigration, with 36 per cent favouring enforced repatriation. The second figure rose to 40 per cent among the over-65s (*Sunday Express*, 27 September 1993). This poll was conducted after the BNP by-election success, and therefore some responses must have been based on the media coverage that it received and not on the true facts about immigration mentioned above, namely that in the 1990s, no large-scale immigration of Asians and other non-whites is taking place. The BNP candidate was defeated by the Labour Party candidate at the 1994 local elections and, therefore, in Britain there are now no elected representatives of the National Front or the BNP. Both the thirteen BNP and the fourteen National Front candidates at the 1992 general election highlighted race and immigration as issues. The Conservative Party also used the 'race and immigration' card towards the end of the election campaign when they realised that they were behind in opinion polls. Statements on immigration were made by some senior Conservatives, including the Home Secretary and the Foreign Secretary. The Home Secretary was quoted as saying that the Labour Party would open the floodgates and he also feared that this would ignite a revival of fascism in Britain (*Daily Express*, 7 April 1992). It appears that such statements might have helped the Conservatives to get some extra white votes and possibly lose some ethnic minority votes. Since there were more seats with smaller majorities than usual, this seems to have benefited the Conservative Party electorally.

It appears from the above analysis that the British public and political reactions to South Asian and other non-white immigration were more vigorous and ongoing than they had been to the previous waves of immigration. Signs such as 'All blacks go home' and 'Send them back' as well as 'Paki bashing' and other anti-immigrant activities through leaflets, speeches and demonstrations, have been common in the last thirty years.

The activities of the National Front, the BNP and the BCSI have been prime examples in this context. There are also thousands of racial attacks and racial harassment cases which take place every year. For example, a recent Home Office study showed that there were 130,000 racially motivated reported criminal incidents in 1993. Of these 32,500 were assaults, 52,000 were threats and 26,000 involved vandalism. The study also showed that one in five Asians living in inner-city areas felt that racial attacks were a 'very big' or 'fairly big' problems (*Guardian*, 11 February 1994). This is not the true picture of racial harassment and attacks, because a lot of people in fact do not report such incidents to the police, some believing that no action would be taken by the police. However, the number of cases reported to the police is also increasing. For example, in 1989, the cases reported to the police in Britain were 5,420 and this number increased to over 10,000 in 1994 (Skellington 1996). Research has shown that racial attacks affect Asians more than some other ethnic groups. The Commission for Racial Equality (CRE) revealed in 1993 that 49 per cent of victims of racial attacks were Asian, 23 per cent Afro-Caribbean, 22 per cent white and 7 per cent Jewish (CRE 1993). In addition there are thousands of acts of racial discrimination which Asians and other ethnic minorities face every day because of their colour and religious and cultural backgrounds.

The political and public reactions to Asians and other non-whites in Britain made them both aware of the dangers and concerned about their insecure position in society. As a response to these dangers, they also started forming organisations to counter anti-immigrant propaganda and highlight the facts of racial prejudice and discrimination. The Standing Conference of West Indian Organisations was formed in 1960 after the Notting Hill riots and the Indian Workers Association, which was formed as far back as the 1930s, also became active from the 1960s. To fight racial discrimination and racial disadvantage, some multi-ethnic organisations were also formed. Among these, the Campaign Against Racial Discrimination (CARD) was set up in December 1964, to influence central government, Parliament and the media to 'build a mass united front for coloured immigrants and their children'. However, due to various tensions about the two roles and between the West Indians, Indians, Pakistanis and white British, the organisation collapsed after three years (Heineman 1972). In February 1965, the Racial Adjustment Action Society was formed, and in June 1967, the Universal Coloured People's Organisation was set up. These organisations were joined mainly by West Indians. South Asians also set up various social, welfare and religious organisations at national and local levels. It is worth pointing out here that, from the early 1960s, several attempts have been made in Britain to set up organisations which include all ethnic minorities. However, this effort has not been successful over a long period, although on certain issues of common concern some such organisations were formed, even in the early days of migration. For example, in 1961, a Committee of Afro-Asian Caribbean Organisations was set up to oppose what became the 1962 Act when it was going through Parliament. Another opportunity for non-whites to participate in policy implementation was provided through the National Committee for Commonwealth Immigrants (NCCI) in 1965, set up like the RRB as a result of the first Race Relations Act 1965. The NCCI was replaced in 1968 by the CRC. This was followed in 1970 by the setting up of the United Kingdom Immigrants Advisory Service (UKIAS) to assist with appeals by those who were refused entry to the United Kingdom. More recent multi-ethnic organisations to fight increasing racism include the Anti-Nazi League and the Joint Committee Against Racialism (JCAR), formed in 1977, and the Anti-Racist Alliance (ARA), launched in 1991. In addition some national Asian organisations currently exist, including the Standing Conference of Pakistani Organisations (SCOPO), the Confederation of Indian Organisations and the Federation of

Bangladeshi Organisations. There are also several national minority religious organisations, which include the Union of Muslim Organisations (UMO), the UK Islamic Mission, the Supreme Council of Sikhs and several Hindu organisations. Some Asian professional and business organisations have also been formed to meet the needs of their members, including the Overseas Doctors' Association (ODA), which is dominated by Asians and in fact is now twenty-one years old. Most of these organisations are helping their members to get equality, among other objectives (see also Chapter 11).

STRUCTURE OF THE BOOK

Chapter 2 deals with the settlement patterns of South Asians in Britain and describes their demographic and religious characteristics. Chapter 3 analyses the various aspects of education of young Asians and how these compare with white young people by using empirical data from the surveys. It also examines teachers' attitudes, in particular, to racial stereotypes and racial discrimination. In Chapter 4 the career aspirations and experience of young Asians in the labour market are examined and are also compared with those of white young people. Chapter 5 analyses the housing situation of Asians and presents the views of young Asians, and Asian parents about living in Asian concentration areas, and their reactions to the extent of racial discrimination in housing. In Chapter 6 the experience and attitudes of young Asians and Asian parents regarding racial violence and harassment, and their attitudes towards race relations, are presented.

Chapters 7, 8 and 9 deal with the religio-cultural issues by using empirical data. Chapter 7, for example, looks at the family and the institution of marriage, Chapter 8 covers the various religious aspects and the question of the mother tongue, and Chapter 9 analyses the attitudes of young Asians and Asian parents towards the issues of leisure, freedom and clothes. In Chapter 10 the responses of policy makers and professionals to the situation of young Asians are presented. Chapter 11 focuses on Asian communities' responses to the needs of young Asians and their participation in the political process. Finally, Chapter 12 draws conclusions about the position of young Asians in British society and their responses to religio-cultural issues.

Chapter 2

Settlement patterns and characteristics

Most Asian workers were economic migrants and they filled a gap for labour mostly in the unskilled sectors and poorly paid jobs, as a result of the reconstruction and expansion of British industry after the war. Their position in the labour market is a fundamental aspect of their position in British society. The type of work available to them on arrival did not merely govern their incomes, it also determined in which areas they settled, where their children went to school, their chances of participation in civic life and their overall status in society. Since they were granted access only to a limited range of occupations upon arrival or through the voucher system, as a consequence there were, and still are, concentrations in certain industrial sectors and factories, and this partly helps to explain their concentration in certain towns, cities and regions of Britain. Kinship and friendship networks also played an important part in this process of concentration. As a result the Asian population is not distributed throughout the country in the same way as the white population. A large number of Asians and other ethnic minorities live in a small number of local authority areas and there is a further concentration of them in a small number of parliamentary constituencies and electoral wards (Anwar 1994). The overall pattern of settlement has not changed significantly in the last twenty years.

SETTLEMENT PATTERNS

The 1991 Census showed that out of the 54.9 million total population of Britain, the ethnic minority population was just over 3 million (5.5 per cent). The census also showed that most of the ethnic minorities were to be found in the south east (56.4 per cent)

Table 2.1 Ethnic minorities in Britain by region, 1991

Regions and metropolitan counties (MCs)	Total population (000s)	White			Ethnic minorities		
		000s	%	% British population	000s	%	% of British population
South east	17,208.5	15,513.8	90.2	29.9	1,694.7	9.8	56.4
Greater London	6,679.7	5,332.9	79.8	10.3	1,346.8	20.2	44.8
East Anglia	2,027.0	1,983.7	97.9	3.8	43.3	2.1	1.4
South west	4,609.6	4,546.9	98.6	8.8	62.7	1.4	2.1
West Midlands	5,150.1	4,727.2	91.8	9.1	422.9	8.2	14.1
West Midlands MC	2,551.7	2,179.2	85.4	4.2	372.5	14.6	12.4
East Midlands	3,953.3	3,764.5	95.2	7.3	188.8	4.8	6.3
Yorkshire & Humberside	4,836.4	4,621.2	95.5	8.9	215.2	4.5	7.2
South Yorkshire	1,262.6	1,226.0	97.1	2.4	36.6	2.9	1.2
West Yorkshire	2,013.7	1,848.6	91.8	3.6	165.1	8.2	5.5
North west	6,243.6	6,000.4	96.1	11.6	243.2	3.9	8.1
Greater Manchester	2,499.4	2,351.9	94.1	4.5	147.5	5.9	4.9
Merseyside	1,403.6	1,378.3	98.2	2.7	25.3	1.8	0.8
North	3,026.8	2,989.0	98.8	5.8	37.8	1.2	1.3
Tyne & Wear	1,095.2	1,075.5	98.2	2.1	19.7	1.8	0.7
Wales	2,815.1	2,773.9	98.5	5.4	41.2	1.5	1.4
Scotland	4,998.5	4,934.5	98.7	9.5	64.0	1.3	2.1
Britain	54,860.2	51,843.9	94.5	100.0	3,006.5	5.5	100.0

Source: 1991 Census

especially in the Greater London Area (44.8 per cent), the Midlands (20.4 per cent), the north and north west (9.4 per cent), and Yorkshire and Humberside (7.2 per cent), with the remainder (7 per cent) in East Anglia, the south west, Wales and Scotland, mainly in Glasgow and Edinburgh. Table 2.1 gives the details.

The census showed that out of the ethnic minority population of just over 3 million, almost half (49.1 per cent) were of South Asian origin, about 0.89 million (29.5 per cent) were black and the remaining 21.4 per cent were Chinese or originated from other parts of the New Commonwealth, as presented in Table 2.2.

Table 2.2 Ethnic minority groups in Britain, 1991 (thousands)

Ethnic group	Britain	England and Wales	England	Wales	Scotland
White	51,843.9	46,907.8	44,114.6	2,793.3	4,936.1
Black Caribbean	499.1	499.0	496.3	2.7	0.0
Black African	207.5	205.5	203.2	2.3	2.0
Black other	178.8	176.4	172.9	3.5	2.4
Indian	840.8	830.6	823.9	6.7	10.2
Pakistani	475.8	454.5	448.8	5.8	21.2
Bangladeshi	160.3	159.5	156.1	3.4	0.8
Chinese	157.5	147.3	142.4	4.9	10.2
Other Asian	196.7	193.2	189.7	3.5	3.5
Other	290.1	281.0	273.3	7.7	9.2
Total population	**54,860.2**	**49,861.6**	**47,026.5**	**2,835.1**	**4,998.6**
Ethnic minority population	3,006.5	2,947.0	2,906.5	40.5	59.5
Ethnic minority population %	5.5	6.0	6.3	1.4	1.3

Source: 1991 Census

Indians are the largest (1.5 per cent) ethnic minority group identified by the 1991 Census, followed by Black Caribbean (0.96 per cent) and then Pakistani (0.91 per cent) ethnic groups. Black African and Black other form 0.7 per cent of the total population, while Bangladeshi (0.3 per cent), Chinese (0.3 per cent), Other Asian (0.5 per cent) and other ethnic groups make up the rest of the ethnic minority population in Britain.

Because our concern in this chapter is with the settlement pattern of South Asians, their regional distribution is presented in Table 2.3.

Table 2.3 South Asian population in regions, 1991 (thousands)

Region	Indian	Pakistani	Bangladeshi	Total
South east	445	143	104	692
East Anglia	7	6	2	15
South west	11	4	2	17
West Midlands	159	99	19	277
East Midlands	99	18	4	121
Yorkshire & Humberside	41	95	8	144
North west	56	77	15	148
North	8	9	4	21
Wales	6	6	4	16
Scotland	10	21	1	32

Source: 1991 Census

It is clear from Table 2.3 that all three South Asian groups have some differences in terms of their settlement. For example, Indians are more widely spread but relatively concentrated in the south east and Midlands regions. On the other hand, Bangladeshis are mainly concentrated in Greater London, West Midlands Metropolitan County and Greater Manchester. However, Pakistanis, unlike Indians and Bangladeshis, are less concentrated in the south east and are found in greater numbers in the West Midlands, Yorkshire and Humberside and the north west, but also in Scotland (see Table 2.4). This pattern is linked to their migration process.

Within these regions, as mentioned above, there are further concentrations of Asian groups. Therefore, the 1991 Census information is used here to find the local authority areas with the most prominent Asian groups. The ten areas in which the percentage of all residents of Asian groups is largest are presented in Table 2.5 (Owen 1994).

It is clear from Table 2.5 that the percentage of Indians in the total population of Leicester, Brent, Harrow, Ealing, Hounslow, Newham, Slough, Wolverhampton and Redbridge was over 10 per cent. But for Pakistanis, no local authority area except Bradford (10 per cent) had 10 per cent or over of the population. The same applies to Bangladeshis; except Tower Hamlets (23 per cent), no area had even 5 per cent of the population which belonged to this ethnic group. However, if all three South Asian groups are aggregated, then their composition in several local authority areas becomes significant.

Table 2.4 Regional distribution of Asians, 1991 (percentage)

Regions or metropolitan county (MC)	Percentage of resident population				
	Entire population	Indian	Pakistani	Bangladeshi	Other Asian
South east	31.4	52.9	30.1	64.5	72.1
Greater London	12.2	41.2	18.6	54.2	56.9
East Anglia	3.7	0.8	1.1	0.8	1.7
South west	8.4	1.3	0.7	1.7	2.2
West Midlands	9.4	18.7	21.0	12.2	5.4
West Midlands MC	4.7	16.7	18.8	11.1	3.9
East Midlands	7.2	11.7	3.5	1.8	3.6
Yorkshire & Humberside	8.8	4.8	19.9	5.1	3.5
South Yorkshire	2.3	0.5	2.7	0.8	0.6
West Yorkshire	3.7	4.1	16.9	3.8	2.0
North west	11.4	6.6	16.5	10.4	4.4
Greater Manchester	4.6	3.6	10.5	7.8	2.5
Merseyside	2.6	0.3	0.3	0.9	0.7
North	5.5	1.0	1.7	2.0	1.3
Tyne & Wear	2.0	0.5	0.7	2.0	0.6
Wales	5.1	0.8	1.2	1.9	1.8
Scotland	9.1	1.2	4.7	0.0	2.8

Source: 1991 Census

Table 2.5 Highest concentrations of South Asian groups in local authorities (LAs), 1991 (estimated percentage of total population)

LA	Indian	LA	Pakistani	LA	Bangladeshi
Leicester	22.3	Bradford	10.0	Tower Hamlets	23.0
Brent	17.2	Pendle	9.4	Newham	3.8
Harrow	16.1	Slough	9.1	Camden	3.5
Ealing	16.1	Birmingham	7.0	Luton	2.7
Hounslow	14.3	Waltham Forest	6.3	Oldham	2.4
Newham	13.0	Luton	6.2	Westminster	2.3
Slough	12.5	Newham	6.0	Hackney	1.8
Wolverhampton	11.4	Blackburn	6.0	Islington	1.6
Redbridge	10.2	Rochdale	6.0	Haringey	1.5
Sandwell	8.0	Hyndburn	5.0	Birmingham	1.3

Source: 1991 Census

This information shows that, while the regional pattern does not change to a great extent, there are variations within some regions.

For example, in addition to Tower Hamlets (inner London), several outer London boroughs have significant number of Asians. Outside London, this applies to Leicester, Slough, Birmingham, Manchester and Wolverhampton, among others. Further analysis of the ward-level data suggests that Asians are mainly concentrated in inner-city areas. This type of concentration has clear implications for their education, employment and housing. Therefore, a brief analysis of some relevant Census information about the characteristics of various Asian groups is presented below to put the survey and other empirical material used later in the book in a proper context.

CHARACTERISTICS OF ASIAN GROUPS

Asians in Britain are not a homogeneous group and it is, therefore, very important to describe their similarities and differences in order to understand the empirical evidence about their position in the society and their religio-cultural attitudes and practices presented in other chapters of the book. Some general characteristics of South Asians are presented above. In this section we look at their gender, age, household and family structure, socio-economic status, religious group compositions and the emergence of the second generation.

There was a great imbalance between the sexes in the early period of migration, particularly for Pakistanis (including Bangladeshis). The almost all-male nature of the Pakistani migration was partly due to cultural factors and partly because of the traditional migratory paths developed in the original emigrant areas of Mirpur, Jehlum, Campbellpur in West Pakistan and Sylhet in East Pakistan. In 1961, it was estimated from the 1961 Census that there were 5,380 Pakistani males for every 1,000 Pakistani females. For Indians, the pattern was fairly similar; both Sikh and Gujarati Hindu men came first but started bringing their families over to Britain as soon as discussions about immigration control started in 1959 and 1961. Therefore, the sex ratio for Indians was 1,568 males for 1,000 females. For the total population, it was 937 males per 1,000 females (1961 Census). This gender imbalance in the process of migration is consistent for international migration, which shows that men migrants first establish themselves economically and then bring their families to the new adopted country.

The 1991 Census shows that overall the balance of sexes for ethnic minorities is now corrected (1,001 males to 1000 females).

However, there are variations between ethnic groups. For example, there are more black women than men, as is true for the white population, but there is still a relatively high ratio of males to females among South Asians, particularly among Pakistanis and Bangladeshis (1,063 and 1,091 males respectively to 1,000 females). This is linked to their late migration and partly to the tradition of women staying behind with the joint family. It appears from the trend in the last three decades that, over time, with the arrival of the remaining dependants from Pakistan and Bangladesh, the sex ratio should be moving towards that of the rest of the population.

The South Asian population is much younger than the white population. It has far fewer older people aged 65-plus (2.99 per cent) than does the whites population (16.8 per cent). On the other hand almost 36 per cent of South Asians are under 16 years old, compared with 19 per cent whites (OPCS 1993). However, further analysis shows that there are clear differences between Indians on the one hand (which includes most of the East African Asians) and Pakistanis and Bangladeshis on the other. For Indians, the figure for under 16 was 29.55 per cent, but for Pakistanis and Bangladeshis in the same age category, it was 42.65 per cent and 47.23 per cent respectively. (See Table 2.6 for details of other age groups.) At the other end of the scale, Indians aged 65-plus make up 4.06 per cent, compared with only 1.73 per cent Pakistanis and 1.20 per cent Bangladeshis in this age range. The differences between Indians and the other two Asian ethnic groups can be explained in terms of their longer stay in Britain, but also, as stated above, Indians include most of the East African Asians who migrated as extended family units, including those now in the 65-plus age group.

Table 2.6 Age composition of Asians and whites, 1991 (percentages)

Age group	Indians		Pakistanis		Bangladeshis		Whites	
	Male	Female	Male	Female	Male	Female	Male	Female
0–4	8.9	8.7	13.0	13.3	14.6	15.6	6.7	6.0
5–15	20.9	20.5	29.6	29.5	32.2	32.2	13.8	12.2
16–24	15.0	15.4	16.9	18.0	16.8	18.5	13.0	12.1
25–44	33.8	35.4	24.6	27.1	18.0	23.1	29.8	28.2
45–59/64	17.3	13.3	13.9	9.2	16.9	9.0	22.8	16.6
Pensionable age	4.1	6.6	2.1	2.9	1.6	1.6	13.9	24.8

Source: 1991 Census

The younger age profile of Asian groups has clear implications for their disproportionate needs for pre-school and school education. It also shows that, although their overall population is small, the number of Asian young people is proportionately quite large and is increasing. The increasing number of dependent children also shows that there are clear differences between South Asians as a group and whites, but significant differences also exist between Indians, Bangladeshis and Pakistanis. For example, according to the 1991 Census, the child dependency rate for whites was 31.6 per cent but for all South Asians it was 59.2 per cent, which is almost double the rate for whites. However, the Bangladeshis had one of the highest child dependency rates, at 92.3 per cent, among all ethnic groups, followed by Pakistanis at 77.7 per cent. Therefore, the Bangladeshi child dependency rate is almost three times the rate for whites. This means that, for Pakistanis and Bangladeshis, there are a lot more children in proportion to the population of working age (Owen 1993). At the other end of the scale, the elderly dependency rate for these two groups is only 4.5 per cent and 3.1 per cent respectively, compared to 32 per cent for the white population.

With the increasing number of Asian children, it is relevant to point out here that most of these children are now British-born. This trend is changing not only the composition of various Asian groups but also their nature, where a majority of them are born and or grown up in Britain. For example, 42 per cent of the Indians in Britain, 50.5 per cent of Pakistanis and 36.7 per cent of Bangladeshis were born in the country (OPCS 1993). This ratio of the population born in Britain is likely to increase significantly in the next few years. This emergence of the second generation of British-born Asians is therefore quite clear and significant.

The tendency among all three Asian groups remains towards living in a joint and extended family system as far as possible. This is explained by many Asians as necessary but also as continuing religious and cultural traditions. Family plays an important role in the lives of South Asians. It also helps to continue links with relatives back home. It is not possible to give precise qualitative information about the nature of Asian families in Britain, because such a question was not asked in the 1991 Census, although from various studies we know that a significant number of joint and extended families exist in Britain. However, the 1991 Census provides relevant information about household size, which in some cases reflects the type of family because many Asians do

not distinguish between a household and a family. (For the Census
one person is asked to complete the form on behalf of all members
of the household.) Bangladeshi households were the largest, with a
mean household size of 5.3 compared with Pakistani (4.8), Indian
(3.8) and white (only 2.4). This is partly because Bangladeshi
households include on average a large number of dependent children aged 0–18, i.e. 3.4 dependent children, compared to an average of 3 for Pakistanis, 2.1 for Indians, and only 1.8 for whites. The
1994 PSI survey (Modood *et al.* 1997) also shows that Asian
households were larger than white: Indian (3.9), Pakistani (5.1),
Bangladeshi (5.7) and white (2.4) dependent children per household. A 10 per cent sample of the 1991 Census also provides details
about married couple families on an ethnic basis and those families
with dependent children. Table 2.7 gives the details of family type
for the three Asian groups and for whites.

Table 2.7 Family type with dependent children, South Asian groups and
whites, 1991 (percentages)

Family type	Indian	Pakistani	Bangladeshi	White
Married couple	89.6	86.8	86.4	79.2
With no dependent children	20.6	13.4	8.2	35.6
With one or more dependent children	58.8	68.0	75.1	25.0
Lone-parent families	5.4	9.0	12.0	12.8

Source: 1991 Census

It is clear from Table 2.7 that, amongst Asian groups, Indians
had the highest percentage of married couples, almost 90 per cent,
compared to Pakistanis (86.8 per cent) and Bangladeshis (86.4 per
cent). Compared with whites, the Asian groups show very striking
comparative differences when we look at families with no dependent children (35.6 per cent white and 17.5 per cent Asian) and
families with one or more dependent children (25 per cent white,
62.9 per cent Asian). On the other hand, a very small number of
Asian couples cohabit and a small number (10.2 per cent) are one-
parent families with one or more children. This is a striking finding
which is normally not acknowledged within Asian groups. The PSI
Survey (Modood *et al.* 1997) also found that 8 per cent of Asian
families were lone-parent families, compared with 21 per cent white
and 45 per cent Caribbean lone-parent families.

One survey undertaken in 1982 (Brown 1984) also provides useful information about Asian households. It showed that 29 per cent of Asians households had more than five persons compared to only 3 per cent of white households. It also showed that the percentages for households with more than five persons were even higher for Pakistanis (43 per cent) and Bangladeshis (44 per cent). This survey showed too that 21 per cent of all Asian households had more than one family unit (3 per cent more than two families) and that 16 per cent were horizontally extended households, compared with only 4 per cent whites. Horizontally extended families include members who are related to the head of the household other than husband, wife, child or grandchild, or may involve more than one family unit living together. Asian joint and extended families are normally horizontally extended but are also vertically extended, with two or three generations living within the same family. The PSI Survey (Modood *et al.* 1994) also found that, generally, Indians and African Asians were found in small families but Pakistanis and Bangladeshis had large and complex families and households (Modood *et al.* 1997). Some of the reasons for living in a joint or extended family are explained in Chapter 7. We now turn to social class differences for all three Asian groups and, where relevant, compare them with white people. The latest information about social class emerges from the 1991 Census based on a 10 per cent sample. The Census allocates all employed people into six broad categories: (1) professional, (2) managerial and technical, (3) skilled non-manual, (4) skilled manual, (5) partly skilled and (6) unskilled. It appears that more Indians (9.2 per cent) are in the professional category than even whites (4.8 per cent), and 4.9 per cent and 5.9 per cent of Bangladeshis and Pakistanis are also professionals. This can partly be explained by a large number of Asian doctors in the National Health Service (NHS) (Anwar and Ali 1987). It is estimated that almost one third of the NHS doctors are from overseas, mainly from the Indian subcontinent. There is also now a growing number of second generation British-trained doctors and other professionals. At the other end of the scale, 33 per cent of Bangladeshis are unskilled or semi-skilled compared with 27 per cent of Pakistanis and 24 per cent of Indians, but only 21 per cent of whites are in this category. However, the greatest contrast is between Bangladeshis in the managerial and technical class (12.5 per cent) compared to 26.9 per cent of Indians in this category (28.4 per cent whites and 23.3 per cent Pakistanis). It is interesting to point out that for all ethnic groups the number of manual workers has gone down, but there are still striking differences between some Asian groups and whites. For example, the Labour Force Survey has shown that, overall, ethnic minorities have experienced a faster transfer in the last ten years from manual to non-manual occupations, compared with white workers. In 1984–6, 45 per cent of ethnic minorities were in non-manual occupations, and this increased to 57 per cent in 1993 (Department of Employment 1993), while for whites it increased from 46 per cent in 1984–6 to 51 per cent by 1993. For Asians, some of this change can be explained because of the significant growth in the number of self-employed Asians during this period. It is a well-known fact now that almost 50 per cent of retail outlets in Britain are owned and/or run by South Asians. This trend is likely to continue in the near future.

ASIAN RELIGIOUS GROUPS

It was mentioned in Chapter 1 that Asians not only come from different countries and regions but also belong to different religious groups. Almost all Pakistanis and Bangladeshis are Muslims and a significant number of Muslims come from India. It is estimated that almost 850,000 Muslims in Britain are South Asians (Anwar 1993). Two national surveys in 1982 and 1994 showed that 46 per cent and 45 per cent, respectively, of South Asians in Britain were Muslims (Brown 1984; Modood *et al.* 1997). The 1994 survey also showed that, of the remaining South Asians, 24 per cent described themselves as Sikh, 23 per cent as Hindu and 2 per cent as Christian, and 6 per cent either belonged to another religion (1 per cent), or had no religion (3 per cent) or did not answer the question (2 per cent). The 1982 survey referred to above provided a similar pattern, except that it revealed that, of the total Asian population, 20 per cent were Sikhs and 27 per cent Hindus. Both the 1982 and 1994 surveys had a separate category of African Asians which showed that, in 1994, 54 per cent (60 per cent in 1982) of them were Hindus, 20 per cent (11 per cent in 1982) were Sikhs and 17 per cent (24 per cent in 1982) were Muslims. Among Bangladeshis in both the surveys, 2 per cent categorised themselves as Hindus and 1 per cent as Christians.

On the basis of these surveys and by using the 1991 Census information, it is possible to calculate the approximate number of Asian Muslims, Hindus and Sikhs living in Britain. I would like to emphasise that it is approximate because I am writing in 1997 and the Census was undertaken in 1991. Also, there are estimates provided by religious leaders of all three groups which are greater than the estimates provided here. In fact, unless a question on religion is included in a future British Census, as is done in Northern Ireland, it will remain difficult to provide a satisfactory estimate of Asian and other religious groups. However, the precise size of these groups at national level is, in practice, not as important as data about minority religious groups at local level. It appears that currently the Office for National Statistics is taking steps to do a feasibility study for the inclusion of a question on religious affiliation in the next Census in 2001. This is an idea which has widespread support among all Asian groups.

Chapter 3

Education

Education is an important influence, and what a child learns in school may be more or less compatible with what the child learns at home. Asians attach a great importance to education in school and beyond. Therefore, in this chapter we examine various aspects of the education of Asians and how these compare with the education of white people, by using survey data.

TYPES OF EDUCATIONAL INSTITUTION

First, what types of school had Asians attended? Most Asian young people in the sample (72 per cent) had attended comprehensive schools, compared with 67 per cent whites. Another 23 per cent of Asians, compared with 19 per cent whites, attended secondary modern schools, and 7 per cent of Asians and a higher proportion of 12 per cent of whites attended grammar schools. However, a significantly higher proportion of Asians (15 per cent) compared with only 4 per cent of whites stayed on in sixth-form colleges. It appears from the detailed analysis of the data that Asian young people stay at school longer than white young people. For example, the average age of leaving school for Asians was 17 years 1 month, compared with 16 years and 7 months for whites. Despite the stereotypical perception that many Asian girls are forced to leave school early, no gender differences were found. If anything, in some recent interviews conducted by the author, some young Asian people were claiming that Asian girls stay at school longer than boys. One Asian girl explained this:

> It is a great advantage for Asian girls to stay at school longer because they get a chance to improve their lot academically. But

it is also useful for parents to feel that Asian girls are in a
protective environment, particularly in single-sex schools. I go
to a single-sex school and my parents [Muslim] support my idea
of spending longer at school and then going on to further and
higher education.

(Interview 1994)

It appears that, in the 1970s and early 1980s, there were differences between Asian males and Asian females but, in terms of
patterns, they compared well with white boys and girls. For example, the analysis of school leavers' destination data by Bradford
showed that 51 per cent of ethnic minority (mainly Asian) males
remained at school compared with 22 per cent of whites. For ethnic
minority females, the figure was 37 per cent compared with 27 per
cent of whites. A national study confirmed that more Asians were
going on to full-time education following O-levels or CSEs.
Almost seven out of ten Asian pupils stayed in full-time education
after O-levels and CSEs, compared with four out of ten white and
five out of ten Afro-Caribbean young people (Drew *et al.* 1992). A
survey in Birmingham in 1991 showed that a higher proportion of
Asian than of white pupils were staying on in education after the
school leaving age. It showed that 68 per cent Indian, 58 per cent
Bangladeshi, 57 per cent Pakistani and 52 per cent white pupils
stayed on in education (Anwar 1996). This is in order to overcome
some of the educational disadvantage they face in schools. As well,
with the help and encouragement of Asian parents and other family
members, many Asian pupils aspire to higher education. The PSI
National Survey has also shown that a high proportion of Asian
men aged 16–19 were in full-time education compared with non-
Asians (Modood *et al.* 1997). It showed that 81 per cent of Indians/
African Asians and 71 per cent of Pakistani/Bangladeshi men
stayed in full-time education, compared with 43 per cent of white
and 46 per cent of Caribbean men. However, the pattern of women
was fairly similar for Pakistani, Caribbean and white women and
higher for Indian/African Asian women in the sample.

Those Asians who had gone on to further education after leaving
school were asked what sort of educational institution they had
attended. It is clear from our survey data that 36 per cent of Asians
had attended colleges of further education or former polytechnics
compared with 23 per cent whites, and only 3 per cent Asians had
attended old universities compared with 6 per cent whites in the

sample. However, more recent analysis of the university entry data shows that the number of Asians in higher education is steadily growing, although more still attend the new universities (former polytechnics) than the old. Taylor (1976) in a study of Newcastle upon Tyne showed that there was no apparent difference between Asian and white school leavers. He also found that more Asians went into further education. Craft and Craft (1982) found that Asians at all levels of academic performance were the keenest group to stay on to the sixth form. He discovered that even 80 per cent of Asian pupils from working-class backgrounds were opting for sixth-form courses. Furthermore, at the end of the sixth form, Asian pupils were more likely to remain in full-time education, though their A-level results then tended to be lower than those of whites and they therefore opted for polytechnic rather than university courses.

In the last twenty years some studies have put more emphasis on social background and gender differences (Driver 1980; Maughan and Rutter 1986; Parekh 1983; Eggleston *et al.* 1986; Keysel 1988; Drew and Gray 1990) and others on the school effect (Nuttall *et al.* 1989; Smith and Tomlinson 1989). However, because of different methods used to assess the performance of various ethnic groups in schools, no clear picture emerges from those studies about the factor(s) which contribute to the differential achievement of Asians and other ethnic group children. Drew and Gray (1991) looked at ten studies to find answers to this question of the achievement of various ethnic groups. They concluded, 'To date we lack a study with sufficient number of pupils and schools, covering a sufficient range of variables, with a nationally representative sample combining both qualitative and quantitative forms of data gathering that would provide answer to this question.'

EDUCATIONAL ACHIEVEMENT

The educational achievement levels of Asians compared with other ethnic groups have been discussed widely. Lord Scarman (1981), commenting on the Brixton disorders, said, 'disadvantage in education and employment are the two most crucial facts of racial disadvantage. They are closely connected. Without a decent education and the qualifications such an education alone can provide, a school leaver is unlikely to find the sort of job to which he aspired – or indeed any job.' In this context, Asian parents put a great value on educational achievement. The educational achievement of some Asian groups has improved significantly in the last ten years. This has resulted partly from their length of residence and partly from their upward economic mobility. Therefore, we examine the performance of Asian children in education over time.

The Inner London Education Authority (ILEA) studies between 1966 and 1976 found that, in 11+ and literacy surveys, pupils of Indian and Pakistani origin did better on tests of attainment than other 'immigrant' groups and that their performance improved with their length of schooling in Britain. Even then those fully educated in Britain scored almost as well as white indigenous children. In the 1960s and early 1970s the low literacy scores of Asian pupils were due to their recent arrival in Britain. This was the period during which the dependents of Asians who were legally settled in this country were joining them. In Scotland a study showed that on four tests of 'ability', white Scottish children scored only slightly higher than long-stay Asian children. But short-stay Asian children scored the lowest. However, on attainment levels, the mean score of white Scottish children was lower in all subjects than that of long-stay Scottish Asian children (Ashby *et al.* 1970). Haynes (1971) concluded that pupil–teacher attitudes were crucial in the process of assessment of potential ability. For example, the higher score of Indian-origin children in a 'higher number of immigrant children school' could be explained by teachers there having a more positive attitude to ethnic minorities. In the early 1970s, Ghuman (1975) found that 'English Punjabi' and white boys had similar scores, but boys educated in the Punjab had much lower scores. He explained this in terms of poor educational experiences and their origin in a rural environment compared with the British urban one. Another study (Essen and Ghodsian 1979), based on the data from the National Child Development Study, indicated that Asian children were the highest scorers among 'second generation' immigrant children. Driver and Ballard (1979) found that, with the exception of English language, Asian pupils at three schools achieved higher average results than did English white pupils attending the same secondary schools. Craft and Craft (1982) also showed in a study of an outer London borough that Asian pupils seemed to be doing as well as and sometimes even better than white students. Following this trend and after examining two school leavers' surveys conducted by the Department of Education and Science (DES) in 1978–9 and 1981–2, the Swann

Committee (1985) concluded that Asian leavers were achieving 'very much on a par with, and, in some cases, marginally better than, their fellows from all groups in the same LEAs in terms of the various measures used'. The Swann Committee had also commissioned the National Foundation for Education Research (NFER) to review the research on the education of pupils of Asian origin. This review also concluded that 'most of the studies point to performance levels on the part of Asians that either match or exceed those of indigenous peers' (Taylor and Hegarty 1985).

However, there are indications that, if nationally representative samples are compared, rather than pupils from the same areas, the picture of Asian pupils' achievement levels is mixed. Some have called it 'the myth of South Asian achievement levels' (Tanna 1990). For example, if the actual process of attainment, as opposed to quantifiable examination results, is compared, Asians seem to be more unsatisfied than white pupils. As pointed out earlier, they also spend longer periods in school to achieve good results. The DES surveys in 1978–9 and 1981–2, referred to above, also confirmed this trend, showing that between 25 and 29 per cent of Asians left school at the age of 17 or 18, compared with only 7–10 per cent of West Indians and 16–17 per cent of others in the same age group. Research has also shown that more Asian than white pupils attempt A-levels more than once. One study showed that 24.2 per cent of Asians retook at least one examination, compared with only 10.8 per cent of whites in this group (Tanna 1990). Based on her research, Tanna (1990) has put forward three possible explanations for this trend, namely: (1) many Asians doing some O-levels as well as their A-levels during their sixth form; (2) teachers' attitudes and streaming; and finally (3) 'poor teaching' and 'bad schooling'. Whatever the debates about the processes involved in the achievement levels of Asians, one fact is clear: as a group they have improved their achievement levels over time, but there are differences between various Asian groups. In 1983/4 our survey showed this trend as presented in Table 3.1.

It is clear from the detailed analysis that Pakistani and Bangladeshi young people were less likely to have formal educational qualifications than Indian and East African Asians. Twenty-seven per cent of the Pakistanis and a high of 51 per cent of the Bangladeshi young people in the sample had no formal qualifications compared with only 15 per cent of the Indians and East African Asians. These differences are partly linked with their backgrounds,

Table 3.1 Educational qualifications of ethnic groups

	Asian %	Caribbean %	Whites %
No formal qualification	21	20	24
CSE Grade 2–5	15	23	20
O-level or CSE equivalent	26	32	26
A-level or higher	24	12	20
Information not given	13	12	9
Size of sample	570	507	423

including social class, and partly with the length of stay in this country. Bangladeshi children, for example, are more recent arrivals than the other three Asian groups. This trend of achievement continued in the late 1980s and early 1990s and also applies to higher-level qualifications. The Labour Force Survey (LFS) 1988–90 showed that only 18 per cent of Pakistanis (16–24 age group) and 5 per cent of Bangladeshis had GCE A-level/equivalent or higher qualifications compared with 33 per cent of whites, 36 per cent of Indians and 41 per cent of African Asians, as shown in Table 3.2.

It is clear from Table 3.2 that there are differences between whites, Indians and African Asians on the one hand, in terms of highest qualifications, and Pakistanis and Bangladeshis on the other hand. It is also worth stressing that 54 per cent of Bangladeshi and 48 per cent of Pakistani young people did not achieve any

Table 3.2 Highest qualifications of Pakistanis and other ethnic groups (16–24 age group), 1988–90 (percentages)

Qualification	White	Indian	African Asian	Pakistani	Bangladeshi
GCE A-Level/ equivalent	26	27	26	15	3
Degree/equivalent	4	6	13	2	2
Higher education below degree	3	3	2	1	0
GCE O-Level/equivalent	30	25	20	18	16
Other	3	5	7	5	10
None	20	22	18	48	54
Never received any education	0	0	1	8	5

Source: Adapted from Jones 1993

formal educational qualification, compared with only 20 per cent
of whites, 22 per cent of Indians and 18 per cent of African Asians
in this situation. There were also gender differences, i.e. more
young Asian women than young Asian men were without educational qualifications.

In London, an analysis of the examination performance of 5,500
pupils from six London boroughs in 1990 showed that pupils of
Indian and Pakistani origin performed better than white, Afro-
Caribbean and Bangladeshi children (*Independent*, 29 October
1991). However, there were significant differences in terms of the
examination achievement levels of the pupils of different ethnic
groups in Birmingham, as presented in Table 3.3.

Table 3.3 Year 11 pupils achieving five or more GCSEs at grades A–C by
ethnic group and gender, Birmingham, 1994 and 1995

Ethnic group	1994		1995	
	Male %	Female %	Male %	Female %
White	34	38	33	38
Indian	37	42	37	42
Pakistani	20	22	16	19
Bangladeshi	32	25	30	22
Afro-Caribbean	13	23	13	22

Source: Birmingham City Council Department of Education

Table 3.3 shows that, apart from Afro-Caribbean male pupils,
the performance of Pakistani pupils in terms of achieving five-plus
GCSE grades A–C was worse than that of all other ethnic groups.
The differences between Pakistani and Indian young people are
quite significant. It is also interesting to note that, except Bangladeshi girls, in all ethnic groups girls were performing better than
boys. Data from another local area, Waltham Forest in London,
show a similar trend in terms of ethnic differences regarding pupil
attainment, as shown in Table 3.4.

Table 3.4 shows the continued higher achievement of Indian
pupils, followed by Pakistani and Bangladeshi in 1995. However,
Greek pupils also show a higher achievement in education than
other ethnic groups in the area.

One other way to examine the patterns of educational achievement of young Asians is to look at the qualifications they achieve

Table 3.4 Waltham Forest: pupil attainment survey, 1994 and 1995

Ethnic origin	1994 Survey average GCSE points scored	1995 Survey average GCSE points scored
African	25.6	25.2
Afro-Caribbean	26.7	27.1
Indian	37.7	42.0
Pakistani	33.5	35.1
Bangladeshi	16.9	30.6
White (UK)	29.8	30.0
Irish	33.8	27.2
Greek	37.7	36.8
Turkish	19.2	29.4
Waltham Forest	30.3	31.5

Source: London Borough of Waltham Forest 1996

and their participation in higher education. The 1991 Census gives us the national comparative information with which to look at the qualifications of Asian groups compared with those of whites. Looking at those aged 18–29 with A-levels or better qualifications, it is clear that white young people were less likely to be in this category (21.4 per cent) than Asians (32.5 per cent). Within the Asian group, Pakistanis had higher numbers in this category (39.1 per cent) than Indians (31.4 per cent) and Bangladeshis (25.5 per cent). However, when we look at those in this age group with higher-level qualifications, and compare them with other age groups, a different pattern emerges, as presented in Table 3.5.

The Census information based on a 10 per cent sample return gives us the most comprehensive information on the trend that, on the whole, people of Indian origin are more highly qualified than Pakistanis and Bangladeshis and even whites. This certainly has

Table 3.5 Higher-level qualifications: Asian ethnic groups and whites in Britain, 1991 (percentages)

Age group	White	Indian	Pakistani	Bangladeshi
18–29	12.5	15.2	7.2	3.4
30–44	19.7	17.0	7.6	6.0
45–pensionable age	14.0	14.7	6.4	6.5
Of pensionable age	6.6	3.8	1.8	1.6
All aged 18 and over	13.4	15.0	7.0	5.2

Source: 1991 Census

implications for the achievement levels of their children. The 1991 Census information also confirms that 16–18-year-olds of Indian origin display higher staying-on rates than Pakistanis, Bangladeshis and whites. For example, over 70 per cent of Indians in this age group stay in full-time education. Pakistanis and Bangladeshis show a lower rate but similar patterns; however, for whites the percentage declines from almost 77 per cent at age 16 to just over 30 per cent at age 18. This pattern is consistent with the analysis presented above, of young Asian people staying on longer to overcome any racial disadvantage or discrimination in the policies and practices of schools or colleges they attend.

RACIAL DISCRIMINATION IN SCHOOLS

In this context, we asked young people in our survey of 1983 how satisfied they had been with the last school they had attended. While a significant majority of both Asian and white young people were very or fairly satisfied, a number of Asians spontaneously mentioned racism as a reason for their dissatisfaction. Two types of complaint about dissatisfaction emerged in the responses. One related to the choice of subject they wanted but were refused, and the other was concerned with personal experience of racial discrimination from some teachers.

Young persons in the survey were asked whether they had felt that there was evidence of racial discrimination in the schools they had attended. Almost 40 per cent of Asian young people felt that there was. It is interesting to note in Table 3.6 that 27 per cent of white young people also claimed that there was evidence of racial discrimination in their schools.

Table 3.6 Racial discrimination in schools

	Asians %	White %
No evidence	60	71
Evidence	39	27
Extent of racial discrimination		
Very serious	4	4
Fairly serious	15	9
Not very serious	16	10
Not all serious	3	4
Size of sample	516	423

Those who thought that there was very or fairly serious racial discrimination were asked what form it took. They replied that it mainly took the form of name calling (32 per cent Asian and 22 per cent whites said this) followed by fighting and picking on ethnic minority pupils. One in five of those who felt that racial discrimination was very or fairly serious mentioned teachers' prejudice generally, and a minority mentioned that teachers have low expectations of ethnic minority pupils. One Asian young person illustrated this:

> There was a teacher who used to pick on coloured children and often used 'black' when he referred to any group of children.

Another gave a particular example of prejudice:

> One teacher did not like a girl who was an Arab and picked on her – told her she should not be in this school – banged her head against the wall.

Another commented:

> Most of the time teachers used to ask questions of white persons, not to Chinese or Asians.

One young white person also gave an example to illustrate his answer:

> We were all being cheeky – but teacher went and smacked a coloured girl, in fact thumped her hard and her parents took her away after that. I actually saw it, it was definite discrimination, she was doing nothing different from all of us.

We also wanted to know whether young people experience discrimination from other pupils and what form it takes. Almost 50 per cent of young Asians claimed to have experienced discrimination from other pupils. This included name calling (27 per cent), fighting (12 per cent), verbal abuse and swearing (13 per cent), teasing, bullying and other forms (14 per cent). One Asian young person explained her personal experience: 'got jumped by skinheads – teachers never did anything'. Another said, 'they called you a "Paki" or a "smelly Arab" when there was a fight'. Several other cases of discrimination by other pupils and teachers were mentioned during the interviews. In fact, the more recent empirical information collected by the author from Birmingham shows that Asian pupils in mainly 'snow-white' areas face more discrimination than do pupils in majority Asian schools. One Asian boy commented on this difference in this way:

> I have a relative in Solihull who goes to a predominantly white school and he has experienced a lot of verbal abuse and has been beaten several times by a gang of white pupils. But, you know, I go to a mainly Asian school in Birmingham, Small Heath area, where white children are more submissive and do not dare to swear at me and abuse me because, you know we are strong and united as Asians.
>
> (Interview 1992)

Parents of young people were also asked about their own experience of racial discrimination in schools. Eleven per cent of Asian parents in the sample had themselves experienced racial discrimination in their child's school. One Asian parent said that, 'Teachers would not let her do what she wanted to do. And about girls regarding physical education they don't understand religious problems.' Another Asian parent talked about his son's experience: 'My son was the first Sikh child to go to school with a turban on and he was attacked physically, tore apart his turban.'

Several examples from Asians regarding discrimination were linked to the questions of religion and culture, and Asian parents saw any lack of recognition or provision of relevant facilities as racial discrimination against them. Teachers were largely blamed for lack of discipline in schools which resulted in Asian children suffering psychologically, physically and, as a consequence, sometimes academically as well. Asian pupils' commitment to academic achievement and discipline has, on the one hand, made them vulnerable to racial harassment at the hands of fellow pupils, but, on the other hand, it has made them more attractive to teachers (Gillborn and Gipps 1996). This brings us to the point where we can examine the attitudes of teachers about some of the issues mentioned both by Asian young people and Asian parents.

TEACHERS' ATTITUDES

It is relevant to mention, first, what types of teacher were interviewed before we look at their attitudes. The schools selected for the 1984 survey were those which had a high, average and low proportion of ethnic minority pupils in the areas covered in the study. Three schools in each area were selected. A cross-section of teachers from different levels of seniority were interviewed, including those who had special responsibilities for careers advice and pastoral care. In total, 85 interviews were obtained with teachers and a majority of the questions were concerned with obtaining their views about racial stereotypes of pupils and parents.

Let us first look at teachers' view of young Asians' performance at school and how it compares with the evidence presented above. Four out of ten teachers thought that Asians do the same as whites in public examinations. However, 24 per cent of teachers believed that Asians do better at public examinations, because of parental pressure to succeed at school and because Asians are more motivated and hard working. The minority (18 per cent) who thought that Asians did worse in public examinations attributed this to language difficulties. A few comments to illustrate these points are as follows:

> Asians are more dedicated to their work. Parental insistence on doing well. They are in an area they have to compete. They want to please the teachers.
>
> (Scale 1 teacher)

> Asian girls are not encouraged by home background to do exams even if they are capable. They know they have no need to get jobs and are not encouraged to get jobs and they miss schooling at important times either because they are sent on long visits to Pakistan or are kept at home. As far as boys are concerned it is the other way around, they are pushed by parents, too much sometimes. If Asian boys are compared with white boys they are the same but some still have poor command of both written and spoken English.
>
> (Pastoral head)

In the context of teachers' opinion of parents, we wanted to know how much interest parents took in the progress of their children at school. Almost half of the teachers thought the Asian parents showed more interest in their children's progress at school than white parents. It was thought that Asians had high aspirations for their children and had strong family ties. Participation by Asians in parents' meetings was also taken as a sign of their interest in their children's progress, as one teacher explained:

> Asians are keener for their children to succeed. When we have a parents' meeting we get more Asian parents proportionately.
>
> (Scale 1 teacher)

A department head gave his reasons for Asians' success in education:

> The family is strong as a unit and they put more value on education.

A careers teacher said:

> I am judging by parents' evenings and from what kids come and say to me. It has definitely been discussed at home what the child should do as career.

All these comments show that now teachers are generally satisfied with the involvement of Asian parents in their children's education, whereas a few years back the lack of their involvement was generally a common complaint.

However, 71 per cent of teachers felt that Asian parents were less involved in the extra-curricular activities of schools than white parents. Only 6 per cent of teachers said that Asian parents were more involved in extra-curricular activities than white. The main reasons given for Asian parents being less involved in these activities were language difficulties (mentioned by twenty-four of sixty teachers saying they were less involved) and because they felt out of place (sixteen mentioned). A quarter of those teachers also thought that Asians were less likely to attend parents' evenings than whites. One teacher commented:

> It is one of the problems we hope to solve next – that Asian parents don't like coming into schools. The environment at most schools, extra-curricular activities contains a large number of cultural disincentives for Asians, e.g. most functions involve gambling even if it's just a raffle, drinking alcohol, meat eating of some kind and these things are frowned on by some Asian groups.

A careers teacher explained:

> School is not really there for social side of life as far as they are concerned.

It appears that some teachers have stereotyped views of Asian young people, about their performance in public examinations and about their parents' involvement in this process and the extra-curricular activities in schools. However, what is also relevant here is the question of what provisions for multi-cultural education were made in schools.

One fifth of all teachers interviewed claimed that there was no provision for multi-cultural education in their schools and 14 per cent claimed that provision was under review. It is worth pointing out that all these schools were in areas of high ethnic minority concentration. The main multi-cultural provision made in the curricular (21 per cent) or extra-curricular activities (11 per cent) is shown in Table 3.7.

Table 3.7 Teachers' views of provision made in school for multi-cultural education

Provision	Teachers %
None	20
In curriculum	21
Have working party/special person to look at this	14
Extra-curricular activities	11
School is multi-racial because of racial mixture	11
In prayers/assembly	9
English as a second language	7
Teach community languages	5
In school meals	1
Other answers	11
Don't know/don't understand term	13

Base: All (85)

It is interesting to note from Table 3.7 that 13 per cent of teachers were either showing their ignorance of, or did not understand, the term 'multi-cultural education'. Some qualitative comments are reproduced below which illustrate various dimensions of multi-cultural education:

The whole nature of school is multi-cultural by its racial composition. If you mean, can they study their own languages then the answer is yes – here they are called country languages. As far as RE is concerned, these aspects are considered and their needs catered for, e.g. special prayers etc. Consideration is given to eating, e.g. Halal meat is provided.

(Head of department)

Opportunities for ethnic groups to make special study or join in cultural aspects of their group, e.g. religious aspects (assemblies), Asian dance, sports activities, music, e.g. steel band.

(Deputy head)

We had a show of their ethnic clothes, we attempted to do dance. The last two periods on a Friday are for minority time activities and we include in that things that the pupils want, like Asian dance. Some ethnic cooking in home economics. There is a feeling amongst a minority that multi-racial character of the school itself was a form of multi-cultural education.

(Teacher)

Multi-cultural studies not taught as such – we do not think about it in such terms – but bring it in without thinking. I teach geography. We deal a lot with underdeveloped countries and take examples from South Asia though rarely from West Indies.

(Senior teacher)

These comments and others show clearly that multi-cultural education is seen by teachers generally as something additional, marginal and not very significant, not, as the Swann Committee implied, 'education for all'. It appears that white students are not seen, on the whole, by teachers as part of multi-cultural education.

In this context teachers were asked whether their local education authority (LEA) had made any specific provision for teaching ethnic minority pupils in schools. English as a second language was the most common special provision made by LEAs (58 per cent of teachers said this), followed by 16 per cent who mentioned mother-tongue teaching, and 12 per cent religious education. Only 5 per cent of the teachers mentioned the teaching of Asian languages. However, a quarter of teachers claimed that no special provision had been made by their LEA for the teaching of ethnic minority pupils. With such claims by teachers, we wanted to know whether they were satisfied with provisions for teaching ethnic minority pupils. As is presented in Table 3.8, just over 50 per cent were extremely or quite satisfied with the existing provisions but 20 per cent were dissatisfied.

Teachers were also asked whether there were any special provisions for careers advice and for advising and counselling ethnic minority pupils on any special problems or difficulties. Surprisingly, the majority of teachers in the sample (60 per cent) claimed that there was no special provision made for careers advice for ethnic minority pupils, although, in a few cases, a careers teacher (40 per cent) or advisor (11 per cent) was given special responsibility for ethnic minority pupils. Also, an overwhelming majority of

Table 3.8 Teachers' satisfaction with provisions for teaching ethnic minority pupils

Level of satisfaction	%
Extremely satisfied	9
Quite satisfied	42
Neither satisfied nor dissatisfied	21
Quite dissatisfied	16
Extremely dissatisfied	4
Don't know	7

Base: All (85)

teachers (92 per cent) claimed that there was only one advisory and counselling service for all pupils, with no special service for ethnic minority pupils. It is relevant to note that 55 per cent of the teachers admitted that the special needs of ethnic minority pupils might not be catered for by this service. The other teachers felt that the staff were sensitive to the problems of ethnic minorities and were aware of the difficulties which might arise because of cultural differences. Asian girls were mentioned as a group which might be more likely to need special attention. A head teacher commented:

> I think there is an understanding of the special problems likely to face Asian children as they are aware of problems of other children. All children have their own problems and we like to treat them as individuals and Asian girls may have problems specific to themselves. We are conscious of career and marriage problems of Asian girls.

Teachers were also asked what other provision could be made in their schools for Asian and other ethnic minority pupils. The answers varied a lot, with the most commonly mentioned facilities being mother-tongue teaching (18 per cent), a more multi-cultural curriculum (13 per cent), special meals (11 per cent), English as a second language (8 per cent), religious education (8 per cent), and changes in the curriculum to make the contents more relevant to ethnic minority pupils.

Another question was asked towards the end of the interview to check teachers' opinions of what policies and practices were generally needed to meet the requirements of a multi-racial, multi-cultural school. Twenty-four per cent of the teachers saw a wider, multi-cultural curriculum as being needed, followed by 22 per cent who thought recognition of different religious beliefs and cultures was important. Other suggestions made by teachers are shown in Table 3.9. One interesting suggestion in the table is the recruitment of teachers of different races.

Table 3.9 Teachers' opinions of policies and practices needed to meet the requirements of a multi-racial, multi-cultural school

Policies and practices	%
Wider/multi-cultural curriculum	24
Recognition of different religion, beliefs, cultures	22
Equal treatment but certain groups getting special attention if necessary	18
Better training for teachers	18
English-language teaching	16
Teachers of different races	16
Making white children aware of problems of ethnic minority children	8
Teachers developing links with communities	8
Awareness of racism	6
Developing positive self-image for ethnic minorities	5
Better counselling procedures	4
Better school–home liaison	4
Spending more time with pupils/parents	2
Appointment of sympathetic staff	2
Other answers	22

Base: All teachers (85)

We look next at the teachers' attitudes to the recruitment of teachers from ethnic minorities. The results showed that two-thirds of them (68 per cent) believed that efforts should be made to recruit more teachers from ethnic minorities, with 26 per cent not in favour of this, and 6 per cent not knowing. It is worth pointing out here that 92 per cent of the respondents were white, 2 per cent Asian, 1 per cent West Indian and 5 per cent others. The main reason put forward for the recruitment of more ethnic minority teachers was that schools would then represent the make-up of the community. The main advantages for ethnic minority pupils in this context were that the ethnic minority teachers would be more understanding and sympathetic (39 per cent of the teachers mentioned), and act as role models with whom the pupils could identify (35 per cent). A quarter of the respondents also mentioned the fact that teachers, parents and pupils would share a common language. Some illustrative comments are presented:

> Advantage as a role model. He may understand certain problems that they have – some may feel more at ease with them. They may be more aware of certain biases in our education, such as history, literature, etc., and be able to point them out.
>
> (Scale 1 teacher)

> In a multi-cultural school there is a strong argument for a multi-cultural staff but they must be there on merit. Advantages are to identify and understand cultural problems.
>
> (Head teacher)

> From a language point of view, many parents and pupils have language problems so this disappears with a teacher from the same background. Also these teachers can act as interpreters. Asian teachers also understand cultural backgrounds better, e.g. they understand upbringing of girls which I myself can't understand at all... understand attitudes of parents to girls' in jobs. Parents either don't want to talk to me or feel it is none of my business to look into these things but they will talk to Asian teachers.
>
> (Careers teacher, scale 4)

It is worth pointing out that only a minority of the respondents (16 per cent) believed that there would be no advantages in having teachers of ethnic minority origin. However, other surveys have shown that ethnic minority teachers are under-represented in the profession. For example, one survey, conducted in eight LEAs with ethnic minority concentrations, showed that only 2 per cent of the teachers were of ethnic minority origin (Ranger 1988). The overall picture showed that ethnic minority teachers were disproportionately on the lowest salary scales, and were concentrated in subjects where there was a shortage of teachers or where the special needs of ethnic minority pupils were involved. With the present trends of ethnic minority students in teacher training and the age profile of current ethnic minority teachers the signs are that, in the short term, the number of ethnic minority teachers is likely to remain low. Local authority data also confirm the low numbers of ethnic minority teachers. In Ealing, where almost one-third of the population was from Asian and Afro-Caribbean backgrounds in the mid-1980s, there were only 200 teachers of ethnic minority origin out of a total of 2,400 (London Borough of Ealing 1988). In Birmingham, where the pupil population of Asian origin in 1994 was almost 30 per cent (in the LEA-maintained schools), the number of Asian teachers was only 3.1 per cent, and reached 4 per cent in 1995, which is still very low.

One issue which emerged from the interviews with Asian parents and young people was the experience of and attitudes towards racial discrimination in schools. Therefore, in our interviews with teachers, we wanted to know about their awareness of racial discrimination in their school and their attitudes towards such behaviour. We also wanted to learn whether racial discrimination was between pupils, between teachers and pupils, between teachers or between parents and teachers.

Over half of the teachers interviewed (55 per cent) were aware of racial discrimination in their schools. It is important to point out that only two teachers said that there was no discrimination between pupils, which shows a serious situation in schools. The most common forms of racial discrimination which took place between pupils was name calling (seventeen teachers mentioned) and verbal abuse (fourteen teachers). Twelve teachers mentioned physical violence between pupils and nine mentioned tension between different religious sects. Graffiti was also mentioned by four teachers. On the other hand, nearly half (twenty-one teachers) of those who were aware of racial discrimination in their school thought that there was no racial discrimination between teachers and pupils. However, a small minority mentioned teachers insulting ethnic minority pupils (nine teachers) and name calling (six teachers). There was some general feeling that racial discrimination between teachers and pupils was difficult to define and may have been due to unconscious attitudes. In this context, two comments, as examples, are relevant to Asians:

It is very subtle. Can be simply in the teachers' attitudes that these people are to be suffered. There are things which give away attitude, e.g. a teacher saying that Asian children never washed their hands. The main problem lies in attitudes of older teachers whose ideas are ingrained. I don't know what happens behind closed doors of classroom. It may be more open there. I have heard pupils mention particular teachers and I am sure they are right because I have seen signs of racist attitudes but is it very difficult to pin down.

(Pastoral head)

Another teacher commented:

> I heard one teacher refer to an Asian pupil as a wog on the phone.
>
> (Scale 1 teacher)

These comments show the prejudice some teachers have against Asians and other ethnic minority groups, and obviously racial prejudice often leads to racial discrimination. As far as racial discrimination between teachers was concerned there was a low level alleged. This is not surprising because so few schools had ethnic minority teachers. However, a minority of respondents (ten teachers) thought that other white teachers sometimes were sarcastic or patronising to ethnic minority teachers. Some believed that ethnic minority teachers had a low status because of the subjects they taught. One pastoral head commented that 'There is a tendency to mock, to denigrate [ethnic minority teachers], that sort of thing – sarcasm.'

A minority of teachers (four out of ten) also said that there was racial discrimination between teachers and parents; that parents complained of teachers who picked on ethnic minority children, and there were misunderstandings due to cultural and language differences. Some mentioned various subtle forms of prejudice and discrimination, as is illustrated by the following comment:

> Have never seen a white parent with Asian teacher so can make no comment about this but white teachers tend to talk down to Asian parents. Also white teachers do not understand home background. White teachers can be impatient and lacking in understanding about such things as religious beliefs, e.g. see right to attend mosques during school time as escaping from lessons. Visits to Pakistan are also seen in the same light rather than used as a teaching aid for geography, e.g. when child returns.
>
> (Scale 1 teacher)

Finally, teachers were asked whether there had been allegations of racial discrimination in their school, and if so, what the allegations were and what action had been taken. Forty-two per cent of all teachers interviewed said that there had been such allegations. These included physical attacks on ethnic minority pupils, compulsory PE where Asian parents did not want this for girls, pupils who were sent back home for wearing national costume, unfair course marks and complaints against teachers, and bias against Asians and other ethnic minority pupils. Teachers gave various explanations of how these allegations were dealt with to the satisfaction of both parents and pupils. However, it appeared from our analysis that 66 per cent of teachers had received no special training for teaching pupils from ethnic minority backgrounds. Those teachers who had had some specific training were then asked whether this had been part of their initial teacher training (7 per cent) or as part of their in-service training (35 per cent). The main benefits mentioned by teachers who had received special training were that it had made them aware of racism and that they were provided with factual information about the religions and cultures of ethnic minorities. One teacher explained:

> Our tutorial group was racially representative and we also had a residential weekend at which four black/Asian tutors from outside the course were present and racism discussed. It made me more aware of my unconscious racism and provided plenty of factual information about background and culture which always helps to fight any prejudice.
>
> (Scale 1 teacher)

On the whole it appears that special training for teachers to cope with a multi-racial pupil population or to reflect it in the schools' educational policies and practices is not seen as a priority by schools. Some of the attitudes reflected in the survey of teachers obviously need to be corrected with training, among other actions. This should be part of initial teacher training, but also special in-service training for all existing teachers seems to be absolutely essential. It appears from our analysis that both young people and teachers particularly, but also some parents in the sample, were aware of racial prejudice and discrimination in schools. This situation could also be tackled by relevant policies and practices in schools to deal with racial prejudice and discrimination, with appropriate sanctions. However, teacher training in this context should also help to make education institutions more sensitive to these issues.

HIGHER EDUCATION

It was mentioned above that Asian young people have a greater tendency to stay in full-time education than do white young people.

More recent information about Asians in higher education shows that their participation is increasing. In 1991, the Polytechnic Central Admission System (PCAS) published its first analysis of the ethnic origin of applicants. It showed that 7.4 per cent of UK-origin applicants were Asians. In 1991, the Universities' Central Council on Admissions (UCCA) also published the ethnic breakdown of applicants. It showed that 8.7 per cent of applicants came from ethnic minorities. Out of these, 53 per cent of white applicants were accepted, compared with 44.7 per cent of ethnic minority candidates (*Guardian*, 13 July 1991). The acceptance level of Asian applicants with two or more A-levels in 1991 was lower than that of whites, as presented in Table 3.10.

Table 3.10 Acceptance rates of applicants to universities with two or more A-levels, 1991 (percentage)

Ethnic group	Acceptance rate
White	54.2
Indian	46.3
Pakistani	40.7
Bangladeshi	44.7
Black African	34.3
Black Caribbean	28.1

Source: Taylor 1992

Table 3.10 shows that Asian applicants, but also blacks, had differential experience in terms of entering universities. The pattern was similar in 1992. In this context, UCCA put forward five reasons for the differential acceptance rates for ethnic minorities (UCCA 1992, 1993; Modood 1993). These are:

1 There are fewer applicants from ethnic minorities for courses with low entrance requirements, such as teacher training courses, which required a 12.6 mean point score for accepted applicants.
2 There are more ethnic minority applicants for subjects such as medicine and law (20 per cent applicants from ethnic minorities), which required a mean score of 26.7 and 25.5 A-level points respectively.
3 Students from ethnic minorities are more likely to apply for a limited number of universities. For example, in 1991, 44 per cent of Asians and 52 per cent of blacks compared to only a third of whites applied to a university in their home region.

4 Students from ethnic minorities were more than twice as likely as whites to have re-sat some or all their examination to get their final grades. Selectors tend to give less weight to qualifications obtained by making more than one attempt.

5 Ethnic minority applicants have a lower average score than whites, as shown in Table 3.11.

Table 3.11 Average A-level scores of applicants to universities by ethnic group, 1992

Ethnic group	Average points score of applicants with two or more A-levels
White	17.8
Indian	16.8
Pakistani	15.4
Bangladeshi	15.9
Chinese	17.3
Black	14.0
Other	17.3

Source: UCCA 1993

Another factor which contributes to the lower acceptance rate of ethnic minority applicants, it appears, is that a significant number of Asian applicants come through further education colleges rather than direct from schools, as compared to white applicants. A further contributory factor is that Pakistanis and Bangladeshis in particular are under-represented at independent schools, and the highest rate of acceptance at universities is achieved by applicants from this sector. Overall, the acceptance rates show that whites were at the top, closely followed by Chinese, with Indians and Bangladeshis 5–10 per cent below, Pakistanis about 15 per cent below, but African and Caribbean applicants 20 per cent and 25 per cent below respectively (Modood 1993). Despite these differences in acceptance rate, and some possible direct and indirect racial discrimination in the higher education system (CRE 1988), the number of Asians in higher education is increasing. For example, the figures from 1994 show that the percentage of Asians in higher education is reflecting their percentage population, as presented in Table 3.12. However, we should not forget that Asians' age profile is much younger and there should be a higher proportion of Asians in higher education institutions than at present to reflect this demographic fact.

Table 3.12 Asians and other ethnic groups in higher education, 1994

Ethnic group	Female	Male	Total	%
White	431,412	410,956	842,368	61.5
Black Caribbean	8,486	4,933	13,419	1.0
Black African	6,690	8,937	15,627	1.1
Black other	2,977	2,239	5,216	0.4
Indian	12,873	14,588	27,461	2.0
Pakistani	4,709	7,928	12,637	0.9
Bangladeshi	323	2,004	3,327	0.2
Chinese	3,885	3,739	7,624	0.6
Asian other	4,229	5,293	9,522	0.7
Other	7,113	7,314	4,427	1.1
Not known	501	523	1,024	0.1
Information refused	47,017	52,060	99,077	7.2
Information not sought	156,901	161,723	318,624	23.3
Grand total	688,116	682,237	1,370,353	100

Source: Higher Education Statistics Agency 1995
All UK-domiciled students by ethnicity.

As far as the number of Asians working in the higher education system is concerned, in 1995, there were 865 ethnic Indians, 178 Pakistanis and fifty-one Bangladeshis out of a total of 114,721. As in the teaching profession, referred to above, very few Asians work in higher educational institutions, and it appears that, like Asian teachers, they are mostly to be found at lower levels and very few in senior positions. For example, a significant number of Asians work

Table 3.13 Responses to AUT questionnaire

Ethnic group	%
White	95.8
Indian	0.5
Pakistani	0.0
Bangladeshi	0.0
Asian other	0.2
Chinese	0.3
Black Caribbean	0.1
Black African	0.1
Black other	0.1
Other	1.2
Refused	1.8

Source: AUT letter, 1995

as doctors in the NHS, but very few are to be found in teaching positions in medical schools, and those who are are generally on the lower grades and junior partners in research teams.

It is relevant to mention that in a recent survey of the Association of University Teachers (AUT), 9,718 members responded and very few Asians appeared, as shown in Table 3.13. It is clear from those who responded to the the questionnaire that the presence of Asians and other ethnic minority members is not very significant. On the whole, this is a reflection of the serious under-representation of Asians and other ethnic minorities in higher educational institutions.

Chapter 4

Employment

The overall pattern of employment for Asians has changed little in the last four decades: they are now more likely than white people to be unemployed. In 1991, the unemployment rate for Asians was about 25 per cent, compared with 8.8 per cent for whites. However, there were differences between Indians on the one hand (13 per cent), and Pakistanis and Bangladeshis on the other (29 per cent and 33 per cent respectively) (OPCS 1993). The more recent Labour Force Surveys also show a similar pattern where, for example, the unemployment rate, in 1993, for whites was 9.5 per cent compared with Indians (15.2 per cent), Pakistanis (30 per cent) and Bangladeshis (27.7 per cent) (Department of Employment 1993). These differences have remained despite an improvement in the employment situation in some regions of Britain. All the available evidence shows that racial discrimination is a contributory factor to these differences. Even graduates and professional people like doctors and teachers face racial inequality (Anwar and Ali 1987; Ranger 1988; Brennan and McGeevor 1990). The 1991 Census also shows that the unemployment rate for Asians with higher-level qualifications was almost double (6.8 per cent) that for whites (3.6 per cent) in the same category. Therefore, although with higher qualifications one's chances increase, racial inequality still remains an important contributory factor to these clear differences.

The majority of Asians were employed in manufacturing industries and an overwhelming majority of them were working in semi-skilled and unskilled jobs (Brown 1984). However, there are now clear differences between Indians and African Asian men on the one hand, who have similarities to whites, and Pakistani and Bangladeshi men on the other hand, of whom two-thirds are still in manual jobs, compared with 52 per cent of Indian, 44 per cent of

African Asian and 50 per cent of white men in this situation (Modood *et al.* 1997). The manufacturing industries have suffered more in the recent recession, thus disproportionately affecting Asians and other ethnic minorities but the 1991 Census shows that the number of self-employed Asians is increasing at a faster rate than that among the white population. For example, almost 21 per cent of the Asians in employment were categorised as self-employed, compared with 13 per cent of whites. However, the Chinese had the highest rate of self-employment, i.e. 27.2 per cent. This trend is likely to continue as more first generation Asians are being made redundant and young Asian people are unable to enter the job market, partly because of fewer jobs being available and partly because of racial discrimination. Many people are now coming forward to complain formally to the CRE about racial discrimination in employment.

AMBITIONS AND ACHIEVEMENTS

It is normally stated by those professionals who deal with Asian young people that Asian parents' ambitions for their children are generally unrealistic. In a survey of Asian parents in 1975, we found that parents wanted better jobs for their children than they actually obtained. It appears from Table 4.1 that many more Asians worked in clerical office work than parents wished (73 per cent against 11 per cent).

Table 4.1 Asian parents' ambitions and children's achievements in relation to work, 1975

	All parents	
	Job desired for child	Job child is doing
Medical professionals	11	5
Engineering (professional)	11	8
Professional white-collar	11	8
Clerical office work	11	73
Unskilled service job	3	16
Family business	3	5
Other	11	11
Left decision to child	24	—
Further education	40	8
Size of sample	349	349

It is interesting to compare Asian parents' aspirations for school leavers in the 1983 survey, which also confirmed the trend, shown in Table 4.2, for more Asian parents and young people to want the school leavers to go on to university education. Professional jobs were the option most favoured by Asian parents and, in the parents' opinions, by their children who were still in full-time education.

Table 4.2 Comparison of parents' own and parents' view of child's aspirations on finishing full-time education

| Aspiration | Asian | | White | |
	Child's wish %	Parents wish %	Child's wish %	Parents' wish %
Further education				
University	26	34	15	12
Polytechnic and other	6	3	6	—
Jobs				
Professional	25	21	21	18
Clerical/office	9	8	1	3
Skilled manual	18	14	18	12
Unskilled manual	1	—	—	—
Other	2	5	21	21
Don't know	15	19	12	26
Sample size	130	130	34	34

Although the sample of white parents is small, the differences between Asian parents' aspirations for their children and those of white parents are interesting. However, here we need to compare these results with the career aspirations of Asian and white young people still in full-time education. Once again this shows, as presented in Table 4.3, that almost half (45 per cent) of the young Asians still in full-time education wanted to go for further education, compared with only 17 per cent of white young people. Almost one in three Asians wanted to go to university, almost four times higher than the percentage of whites. We would now like to compare these aspirations with those of young people who had left full-time education. It appears that their experiences were less fortunate than they hoped. For example, only a small number of Asian young people actually went on to university (1 per cent) or further education institutions (2 per cent). Twenty-three per cent of Asians but also 26 per cent of white young people ended up in

Table 4.3 Career aspirations of Asian and white young people after finishing school, college or university

Aspiration	Asian %	White %
Further education		
University	29	8
Polytechnic and other	16	9
Jobs		
Professional	28	35
Clerical/office	8	1
Skilled manual	9	17
Unskilled manual	2	3
Other (includes sales/retail)	8	9
Sample size	270	96

unskilled manual jobs, compared to the small minority who wanted to do this on leaving full-time education. Details are presented in Table 4.4.

It is worth stressing that some people's memories of what they had wanted at the time showed greater similarities to their actual

Table 4.4 What actually happened on leaving full-time education compared with what was claimed to have been wanted

Experience	Actual Asian %	Claimed Asian %	Actual White %	Claimed White %
Further education				
University	1	4	*	2
Polytechnic and other	2	12	2	6
Jobs				
Professional	3	15	5	19
Clerical	14	15	17	14
Skilled manual	16	21	24	31
Unskilled manual	23	6	26	5
Other (includes sales/ retail)	7	4	2	4
Training scheme	7	—	7	—
Unemployed	11	—	10	—
Can't remember	—	26	—	22
Sample size	300	300	331	331

*Less than 1%.

experiences than what their peers still in full-time education wanted for their future, as presented in Table 4.3. In spite of this, only 6 per cent of Asians and 5 per cent of whites said that they had wanted an unskilled manual job, whereas 23 per cent of Asians and 26 per cent of white young people had actually gone into such work. Similarly, 15 per cent of Asians and 19 per cent of whites had wanted professional work but only 3 per cent and 5 per cent, respectively, had achieved it. Therefore, it is not too difficult to conclude that both Asian and white young people have unrealistic aspirations for some job categories.

We wanted to know what sort of careers advice was given to young Asians and who actually gave this advice to those who were not in full-time education at the time of the interviews. A third of young Asians claimed to have been given no advice on leaving school, compared with 42 per cent of white young people. A substantial minority could not remember any details of advice they had been given. Those who had been given advice were more likely to mention careers advisors and teachers as being the main sources of advice than their parents and family. This finding contrasts with the general view that Asian young people get such advice from their family and friends. The type of advice received is presented in Table 4.5 along with its sources.

Table 4.5 Advice given to Asian and white young people on leaving school

	Asian %	Whites %
No advice given	34	42
Advice given by		
Careers advisors	22	29
Teachers	15	13
Parents/family	8	5
Advice		
Stay on at school	2	3
Another course/further education	24	16
Get a job	17	24
Government training scheme	2	1
Other	3	4
Don't know/can't remember	17	9
Sample size	300	331

Table 4.5 shows that Asian young people are encouraged to go on to further education more than white. Whites are more likely to be advised to get a job. When parents were questioned about the sources of advice on leaving school, it appeared that white parents were more likely (58 per cent) than Asian (24 per cent) to say that parents and other family members had advised their children. They were also much more likely to mention careers advisors (65 per cent) than Asians were (30 per cent). Those whose children had had advice from other people were asked how satisfied they were with the advice given. The majority of Asian parents (68 per cent) and also white parents (54 per cent) were satisfied. However, the parents' main criticism of the advice given was that it was not detailed enough. This was mentioned in particular by white parents (27 per cent), who were perhaps in a better position to comment because of their wider knowledge of the opportunities available, compared with 14 per cent of Asian parents who were critical.

The parents in the survey were also asked how likely they thought it was that their son or daughter would find a job, after completing full-time education. Seventy-one per cent of white parents felt that it was either very likely or fairly likely that their child would find a job, compared with only 39 per cent of Asian parents. The majority of parents who were pessimistic about their child's chances of success blamed high unemployment, and some also mentioned the special difficulties faced by Asian and other ethnic minorities in finding jobs.

Over 76 per cent of Asians and white young people were fairly or very satisfied with their current job. However, a smaller majority, (two-thirds) of Asian parents were satisfied with their children's jobs, compared with 75 per cent of white parents. Whilst the parents and young people considered the nature of the work – whether it was interesting or boring – and the money in deciding why they were satisfied or dissatisfied with the child's job, a selection of other interesting comments is presented below:

Clean job, nice hours, good environment.

(Asian parent)

It is a regular job, I enjoy myself and get along with the people.
(Young Asian)

I am working – lots of people are not working.

(Young Asian)

I did not want her to become a nurse. She is always so tired especially after night shifts. But that is what she wanted.

(Asian parent)

Those Asian young people who were seeking work were looking for skilled manual (24 per cent) or professional jobs (22 per cent) in preference to unskilled manual jobs. However, those young people who were in work tended to be in unskilled manual jobs or in clerical or sales job. In order to conclude whether these young Asians were unrealistic in their aspirations, one would have to look at the vacancies available in the areas at the time of interviews to see if there was a match between the qualifications and experience needed for the jobs that were available and the qualifications held by the young people seeking work. This we were unable to do as part of our research.

UNEMPLOYMENT

We also wanted to know how Asian parents felt about the unemployment of their children. Therefore, those parents whose child was unemployed or on a government training scheme were asked how likely it was that their child would get a job. It appeared that, generally, parents were not optimistic. The 1991 Census also confirms the trend of youth unemployment for the 18–24 age groups for Asians and whites and shows the gap outlined in the survey. Compared with white young people, Asians, particularly Pakistani and Bangladeshi young people, have high unemployment rates, as presented in Table 4.6. For Pakistani and Bangladeshi youngpeople, the unemployment rate was more than double that of white young people, and even for Indian young people, it was higher. Research in this area has shown that racial discrimination is a contributory factor for such wide differences.

Table 4.6 Unemployment among Asian and white young people (16–24), 1991

Indian		Pakistani		Bangladeshi		White	
Male %	*Female* %	*Male* %	*Female* %	*Male* %	*Female* %	*Male* %	*Female* %
25.3	21.0	40.8	35.2	25.1	36.7	18.0	12.3

Source: 1991 Census

In 1982, in a survey of young people (16–20), we found that Asian young people and white young people were equally likely to be employed (Anwar 1982). In both groups, out of every ten young people in the potential workforce, six were in work and four were unemployed. We looked at those in education. There was a big gap between the two groups. The Asians were more likely to be continuing their education (45 per cent) than whites (26 per cent). The question of whether Asians have more difficulty finding jobs than whites thus depends on the extent to which those who stay at school or go to college or university do so from choice or inability to find work. However, there are always area variations. For example, in Birmingham, in 1984, school leavers' figures showed that white school leavers were two and half times more likely than Asians to find jobs. In Bradford, a survey in 1984 showed that only 7.5 per cent of 16-year-old ethnic minority (mainly Asian) job seekers found work, compared with 32 per cent of whites of the same age group (CRE 1985b). In Sheffield, one survey found that only 13 per cent of young blacks were employed, compared with 47 per cent of whites (Clough and Drew with Wojciechowski 1985). Although the overall unemployment rate has generally fallen, in some areas it remains high for Asians and other ethnic minority groups. But there are differences between various ethnic groups. For example, the more recent figures for 16–19-year-olds show that white and Indian/African Asians have unemployment rates of around a third but that over half of the Pakistani/ Bangladeshi and Caribbean young people were unemployed (Modood *et al.* 1997). There is no doubt that racial discrimination is playing its part in the worsening situation of very high unemployment of young Asians of Pakistani and Bangladeshi origin.

It is relevant to mention here that in 1971, the unemployment rate for Asians was just over 6 per cent, compared with 5.4 per cent for the general population, but by 1991, the picture looked very bad for Asians compared with white people, as presented in Table 4.7.

It is clear from Table 4.7 that there are major differences between whites and Asians and between Asian groups as well. For example, Bangladeshi men and women have the highest unemployment rates, followed by Pakistanis. The reason why the figures for Bangladeshi women in both manufacturing and skilled manual categories are either very low or non-existent is because a majority of them have

Table 4.7 Unemployment among Asian and white groups, 1991 (percentages)

	White		Indian		Pakistani		Bangladeshi	
	Male	Female	Male	Female	Male	Female	Male	Female
Unemployment rate	10.7	6.3	13.4	12.7	28.5	29.6	30.9	34.5
Manufacturing (industry)	9.1	7.8	12.7	11.3	27.4	19.2	47.2	5.0
Skilled manual (occupation)	9.6	10.1	13.8	15.3	24.5	27.5	50.0	0.0

Source: 1991 Census

arrived in Britain relatively recently and they are not in a position to look for skilled manual jobs in manufacturing industry. However, when we analyse the unemployment rate for unskilled workers, the Bangladeshi women once again have the highest unemployment rate (28.6 per cent), compared with 5.1 per cent for Indian women and 5.6 per cent for white women in that category. Pakistani women's rate of unemployment in this category was 23.8 per cent. The signs are that, in the short run, the unemployment situation for Asians, in particular for Pakistanis and Bangladeshis, is not likely to improve. Therefore, we need to examine some of the experiences and attitudes of Asians regarding the factors which have contributed to this high level of unemployment or the perceived difficulty in finding jobs.

In our 1982 survey of young people (Anwar 1982), respondents were asked whether it was more or less difficult for people like them to get a job than for other people living in the same area. Asians were more likely to feel it was difficult (39 per cent) than white young people (22 per cent). Respondents who considered finding a job more difficult were asked why they thought this was so. Forty-eight per cent of Asian respondents said that it was because of their skin colour, followed by 15 per cent who said that it was due to employers' prejudice. All the youngsters interviewed were asked to choose a statement on a scale from 'All employers are racially prejudiced' to 'No employer is racially prejudiced'. It is interesting to note in Table 4.8 that one in three Asian as well as white young people chose statements to the effect that at least half of employers were racially prejudiced.

Table 4.8 Perception of employers' racial prejudice

Statement	Asian %	White %
All employers are racially prejudiced	2	1
Most employers are racially prejudiced	11	9
Half are, half are not	23	22
A few employers are racially prejudiced	47	49
No employers are racially prejudiced	6	13
Don't know/no answer	12	6
Size of sample	348	376

Source: Anwar 1982

Unemployed Asians were nearly twice as likely to think that at least half of employers were racially prejudiced (53 per cent) as were those currently in employment (28 per cent). But it is also interesting to note that, in addition to 32 per cent in the first three categories in Table 4.8, another almost half (49 per cent) of the young white people interviewed acknowledged that a few employers were racially prejudiced. In all, 81 per cent of young whites showed their awareness of the existence of the prejudice and discrimination which employers practise against ethnic minorities. When asked if they had ever felt that they were refused a job because of their colour, almost one in four (24 per cent) of employed and nearly four in ten (38 per cent) unemployed Asian young people claimed that they had personal experience of employers' racial discrimination.

RACIAL DISCRIMINATION IN EMPLOYMENT

In the 1983 survey of young people and parents, we repeated the question regarding the extent of prejudice amongst employers, and the responses presented in Table 4.9 show that both Asian and white young people and parents recognise that there were at least a few employers who were racially prejudiced. Those Asians who were looking for work were more likely to think that there were prejudiced employers than those who were in work.

Asian parents are more likely to think that most or about half of employers are prejudiced (43 per cent), compared with Asian young people (28 per cent). This difference could be based on the longer experience of parents in dealing with employers, compared with some young people, who were still in education. This is why we

Table 4.9 Comparison of Asian and white young people's and parents'
attitudes: extent of prejudice amongst employers

	Asian		White	
	Young persons %	Parents %	Young persons %	Parents %
All employers are racially prejudiced	1	*	2	—
Most employers are racially prejudiced	11	10	9	10
About half are racially prejudiced	17	33	15	12
A few are racially prejudiced	45	37	54	53
No employers are racially prejudiced	6	6	10	18
Don't know	21	14	11	7
Size of sample	570	212	427	101

asked respondents about their personal experience of discrimination by employers. Of those who answered the question, one in ten
Asian young people claimed to have experienced racial discrimination personally from employers. Those who were seeking work
were most likely to feel that they had been discriminated against.
Almost four out of ten Asians who had experienced racial discrimination said that it took the form of being rejected at interviews
and one in four complained of condescending attitudes or behaviour. This was particularly a complaint of those who were seeking
work. Although equal proportions of those Asian young people in
employment and those seeking work felt that they had experienced
discrimination, they mentioned different aspects. Those in jobs
were more likely to mention being discriminated against in terms
of promotion, getting pay rises or being allowed overtime, while
those looking for work complained about employers' attitudes and
behaviour.

Asian parents said that racial discrimination from employers
mainly took the form of being given the worst or hardest jobs,
generally being treated badly because of their race or colour, or
name calling. One Asian parent explained:

Always try to get more and hard work from us than whites and
give whites easy and more paying jobs.

The main way that their children had experienced racial discrimination was by being rejected at interview when white children were not. An Asian parent commented:

> She applied for jobs at many places but she could not get a job while all her white class mates are all fixed up with jobs.

As part of our research, we also interviewed forty-six careers advisors and fifty-two job centre workers from the areas covered in the young persons' and parents' surveys. They were asked whether, from their experience, they felt that employers were racially prejudiced against job applicants of ethnic minority origin. Almost 70 per cent of each group felt that a few employers were racially prejudiced. Forty-six per cent of the job centre officials and 37 per cent of careers advisors had received discriminatory instructions at least once from employers in the previous year. We wanted to find out what action was taken after they received such instructions. Two types of action were taken by officers: either to try to persuade the employers to change the instruction or to report the employer to their supervisors. Some admitted (one in six) that, at some time, they had been reluctant to send an ethnic minority applicant to an employer because they thought the applicant might be rejected on grounds of race or colour. Some careers advisors and job centre officials indicated that there was no point in sending people to an employer who would not employ them. Then the officers were asked what action they would take if a job applicant claimed to have been rejected for a vacancy because of racial discrimination. Sixty-seven per cent of careers advisors and 54 per cent of job centre officials said they would report the incident to their supervisor. Thirty-seven per cent of careers advisors and 29 per cent of job centre officials said they would take up the matter with the employer. Also, just over a third of the careers advisors and just over a quarter of job centre officials said they would report the incident to the CRE.

It is worth mentioning here that the careers advisors and job centre officials had guidelines on dealing with discriminatory instructions by employers. When they were asked about these guidelines, 87 per cent of careers advisors and all job centre officials said that they had them. They were also asked whether they had guidelines for circumstances in which job applicants, or they themselves, believed that an ethnic minority applicant had been rejected for a job on the basis of race or colour. Eighty-five per cent of all respondents said that they had instructions for dealing with this sort of situation. However, it is clear from research evidence, and from formal investigations conducted by the CRE in the field of employment, that racial discrimination was widespread at the point of entry in the labour market.

A study in Nottingham between 1977 and 1979 (Hubbuck and Carter 1980) showed that in nearly half of the 100 firms tested, employers rejected Asian and Afro-Caribbean applicants for white-collar jobs in favour of white candidates whose qualifications and job experience were no better. When tests of the same type were conducted nationally by the PEP in 1973/4 (McIntosh and Smith 1974), it was found that the level of discrimination against ethnic minority applicants for white-collar jobs was about one in three. Therefore, the Nottingham survey showed that the rate of discrimination against Asian and blacks was increasing. Ten years later, tests carried out in 1984/5 showed that racial discrimination by employers was as common as it had been a decade earlier (Brown and Gay 1985). The study showed almost four out of ten Asians were not called for interviews, compared with only one in ten white applicants, although their qualifications and experience were similar. Another study in Nottingham in 1994, following the same method as in 1977–9, found that Asian and black job applicants for white-collar jobs were twice as likely to be rejected as whites (Simpson and Stevenson 1994). Therefore, it is clear that a large number of employers still discriminate despite the fact that the first Race Relations Act to tackle discrimination was passed in 1965 – over thirty years ago. Racial discrimination in employment was made unlawful in the Race Relations Act 1968.

It is widely accepted in the Asian communities that finding a job is difficult because of their colour and/or religion and culture. Many of the young people I interviewed in the early 1990s pointed this out clearly. One typical comment was:

> We as Indians, Pakistanis and Bangladeshis are seen a problem as workers. Some employers think we make too many demands about our culture and religion. They sometimes ask you questions about these, that is if they interview you. Many refuse to interview us because they are prejudiced against non-white people.
>
> (Asian young person, interviewed July 1994)

It appears that the perceptions and experience have not changed in the last twenty years. It is interesting to point out that, in our survey of 1975, respondents were asked whether they thought that most Asian people in their area found it difficult to get the sorts of job they wanted. Only 4 per cent of the sample disagreed strongly with the proposition and more than 60 per cent of young people and parents alike agreed. Two main reasons were given: the general nation wide unemployment position and racial discrimination. One Asian young person said, 'factories like English people first and then Asians'. When asked whether they personally had had problems finding the sort of job they wanted, more parents (33 per cent) than young people (22 per cent) said that they had. Some gave racial discrimination as the reason for their problems. When asked directly about racial discrimination, almost two-thirds of respondents agreed that it took place. The feelings about discrimination in finding jobs were common to all sections of the Asian communities, irrespective of national or regional origin, mother tongue or class. One assumption in the early 1970s was that lack of command in the English language was a hurdle for Asian young people in getting jobs. Three-quarters of both Asian parents and young people in the sample believed that employers' assumptions of language problems prevented young Asians from getting the jobs they are able to do. One young person said:

Even if they know the language and have qualifications, still the white people get them.

Another young person felt even more strongly:

I don't think it is the language. It is the racist employers who do not like the coloured to work.

It is clear from the attitudes presented above that Asians feel strongly about the presence of racial discrimination in the employment field and the way it leads to their unemployment or underemployment. We have also shown above that more Asians aspire to professional careers than achieve them. Our evidence also shows clearly that many more young Asians, still in education, hoped to get jobs which their older brothers and sisters had failed to get. It is apparent too that many Asian young people do not live up to the expectations and ambitions of their parents, although there has been some improvement, in the last twenty years, regarding the parents' expectations and the real achievements of Asian young people.

WOMEN

In the 1960s and 1970s, it was accepted that Asian women generally, and Muslim women in particular, had a low level of economic activity, compared with women in the general population. How this situation has changed, both in terms of reality and attitudes to Asian women and work, needs to be examined in an historical context. It was assumed in the 1970s that some Asian women went out to work but many still stayed at home. There were two main reasons why Asian women did not go out to work: (1) for cultural reasons and (2) because some faced language problems. Therefore, in our 1975 survey, respondents were given the proposition: 'The fact that Asian women don't go to work is more to do with their lack of English than with tradition.' Almost 60 per cent of respondents believed this to be true while nearly one third disagreed with it. Agreement with the proposition was particularly strong among Hindus and Sikhs compared with Muslims, the majority of whom disagreed. Details are presented in Table 4.10.

Table 4.10 'The fact that Asian women do not go out to work is more to do with their lack of English than with tradition'

| | All parents % | All young people % | Parents | | | Young people | | |
			Sikh %	Hindu %	Muslim %	Sikh %	Hindu %	Muslim %
Agree	59	60	63	74	42	65	73	46
Neither agree nor disagree	10	13	13	9	9	17	11	13
Disagree	31	27	24	17	49	18	16	41
Base	944	1,117	220	323	358	254	391	426

Source: Anwar 1976

It is clear from Table 4.10 that the differences were religious rather than intergenerational. Basically, it is the Muslim community which took the traditional view. As one Muslim mother said, 'It is because of our religion.' Those who disagreed with the proposition did seem to find language a barrier but saw no alternative. One respondent explained:

When they [Asian women] don't know English they cannot do the work English women do so they feel shy.

When asked what their attitudes were towards Asian girls and young women going out to work, nearly a quarter of the respondents agreed that they should not go out to work. The pattern of difference of opinion was almost the same as in Table 4.10. For example, there was consistent divergence between the views of parents and young people but there were also differences between men and women. There were greater demands from Asian girls (almost 80 per cent) that they should be allowed to work than either their parents (65 per cent) or brothers (60 per cent) would agree to. Once again, religion was the main reason given by those agreeing that Asian girls and young women should not go out to work. Generally, four out of ten Muslims agreed with the proposition, but only one in ten Hindus took this view, with Sikhs midway. One typical answer given by Muslim respondents was based on religious traditions:

> They usually get enough money from husbands working – it is not our custom, women should be in the home.

Another commented:

> Because it is not in my religion that girls go to work when men can do it.

> (Muslim boy)

Some of those who agreed with Asian women going out to work gave financial reasons, and said that women were not earning enough for the family and extra family members needed to work to supplement the family income. However, to find out why Asian women do not go out to work, the proposition was put to respondents that 'More Asian women would go out to work if they did not have to mix with men.' Opinion was divided on this proposition, but generally there was little difference between parents and young people. There were, however, differences between religious groups, and more agreement with the proposition was found amongst Muslims, as presented in Table 4.11.

There was a marginal difference between Muslim young people and Muslim parents but on the whole, in detailed answers given, religious conviction for all groups that men and women should not mix, was the main reason. An additional reason was the personal dislike of many women for working with men.

It is important to stress that, in the 1980s and 1990s, Asian women have been forced to work for economic reasons. However,

Table 4.11 'More Asian women would go out to work if they did not have to mix with men'

| | All parents % | All young people % | Parents | | | Young people | | |
			Sikh %	Hindu %	Muslim %	Sikh %	Hindu %	Muslim %
Agree	38	42	40	30	45	46	27	52
Neither agree nor disagree	18	14	20	17	17	18	13	12
Disagree	44	44	40	53	38	36	60	36
Base	944	1,117	220	323	358	254	391	426

Source: Anwar 1976

the religious differences remain. A national survey in 1982 (Brown 1984) found that Hindu and Sikh women had a higher economic activity rate than Muslim women who were eligible for work. This trend has been confirmed by more recent Labour Force Survey data and by the 1991 Census (*Employment Gazette* 1991; OPCS 1993). At the end of the 1980s the Labour Force Surveys (1987–9) showed that the economic activity rate of Indian women (mainly Hindus and Sikhs) was 58 per cent whereas that of Pakistani and Bangladeshi women (mostly Muslims) was only 21 per cent (*Employment Gazette* 1991). This trend was confirmed by the 1991 Census data which showed that in 1991, while the economic activity rate for Indian women was 55.4 per cent (even higher than for white women, which was 49.7 per cent), the rate for Pakistani and Bangladeshi women was 27.1 per cent and 21.8 per cent respectively.

However, one other factor needs to be mentioned here, which is that a significant number of Asian women, particularly Muslim women, do homeworking, which does not appear in the official statistics about labour market participation. This work is usually done for cultural reasons or because of the need to look after children at the same time. It also helps the family income, although homeworkers are very low-paid and their working conditions are often below normal health and safety standards.

It is important to point out here that the economic activity rate among Muslim young persons is now increasing since a majority of them have gone through the education system in Britain. The most comprehensive figures to look at for this trend are from the 1991

Census. These data show that, in the group of 16–24-year-olds, while Indian young women were relatively more economically active (50.4 per cent), than Pakistani (40.0 per cent) and Bangladeshi young women (32.4 per cent), the difference was not as great as mentioned above for the 16–59/64 age range, i.e. the working-age population. In fact, my recent interviews with both Muslim parents and young people suggest that most of the young Muslim women, with the consent of their parents, look for appropriate work after they complete their education. However, because of widespread discrimination and the lack of enough suitable jobs in the inner-city areas where most of them live, young Muslim women are finding it harder to get jobs. This was also confirmed by a study of Muslim young women in Birmingham (Brah and Shaw 1992), which concluded that whilst some remain opposed to Muslim women going out to work, others hold flexible attitudes on the issue and yet others are positively in favour of Muslim women pursuing their own careers. However, domestic responsibilities, sometimes community pressures, and racial discrimination were contributory factors to a low level of economic activity of Muslim women in the labour market. Therefore, it is too simplistic to explain the low level of labour market participation of Muslim young women in religious or traditional terms. It needs to be seen within the overall position of Asian and other ethnic minority groups in the labour market: that is, they are more likely than whites to be unemployed or under-employed, and those in work often have jobs with lower pay and lower status. This even applies to well-respected professions.

THE PROFESSIONS

A study of doctors (Anwar and Ali 1987) showed that nearly a third of doctors were born overseas (mainly Asian doctors) but only one in six of the total number of consultants and senior house medical officers were from overseas, and that they were concentrated in the unpopular specialities, notably geriatrics and psychiatry. It also showed that, with equal qualifications from the UK compared with white doctors, the overseas doctors wait longer for promotion and that they had to make more applications for posts than their white colleagues. A sample of ethnic minority doctors with all their medical qualifications from the UK confirmed that they faced similar problems to those doctors whose initial medical qualifications were from overseas.

A formal investigation by the CRE into the accountancy profession also discovered that the success rate of white applicants for accountancy posts was nearly three times as high as that of ethnic minority applicants. In addition, from those reaching the interview stage, the white candidates' success rate was nearly twice that of ethnic minority applicants (CRE 1987a). Similarly, a study of career destinations of graduates discovered that those from ethnic minorities (mainly Asians) appeared to experience greater difficulties than whites in obtaining employment (Brennan and McGeevor 1990). A greater proportion of ethnic minority graduates were unemployed twelve months after graduation, and they themselves perceived greater difficulties in gaining employment than did their white counterparts. Ethnic minority graduates continued to have to make more job applications than their white peers. They received fewer interviews, job offers and early promotions, and there was evidence that they were channelled into specific courses and employments which were not seen as prestigious. Asian teachers and other Asian professionals have similar experience of racial discrimination which makes it harder for them to achieve their full potential.

It is clear from the evidence available that tens of thousands of acts of racial discrimination in employment take place in Britain every year and most of the victims have no way of knowing that that is what is happening. High unemployment is hitting Asians harder than whites, and several surveys mentioned above demonstrate that racial discrimination is contributing to this situation and that Asian young people born and educated in Britain are equally victims of this. It is worth pointing out here that discrimination in employment has a magnifying effect on other key areas like education and housing. Therefore, we now examine the housing and social conditions of Asians.

Chapter 5

Housing

As outlined at the end of the previous chapter, it is clear from recent patterns that discrimination in employment has a magnifying effect on other key areas like education and housing. We pointed out in Chapter 2 that Asians generally live in inner-city areas. They face the acute problems of the inner cities and these lead them to suffer an overall pattern of racial disadvantage in housing, in both the public and private sectors. In the 1960s and 1970s, studies looked at the relationship between housing class and class formation (Rex and Moore 1967; Rex and Tomlinson 1979). More recent research has concentrated on tenure patterns and on direct and indirect discrimination by local authorities and the private sector. For example, the CRE's formal investigations into council housing in Hackney and Tower Hamlets in London, together with its research and a formal investigation into council housing allocations in Liverpool, showed widespread discrimination against ethnic minority applicants and tenants (CRE 1984a, 1984b, 1989b, 1989c). The number of individual complaints received by the CRE from Asians and other ethnic minorities against racial discrimination in housing policies and practice are also increasing over time. A report by the CRE, based on testing in thirteen areas in 1990, showed that a fifth of all accommodation agencies consistently treated Asians and other ethnic minority testers less favourably than the white testers (CRE 1990).

HOUSING TENURE, TYPE AND CONDITIONS

The 1991 Census showed that the owner-occupation rate for Asian households was greater (77 per cent) than for whites (66.6 per cent). However, there were differences between Indian, Pakistani and

Table 5.1 Housing tenure of Asians and whites, 1991 (percentages)

Ethnic group	Owner-occupied	Public sector renting	Private sector renting	Rented from housing association
White	66.6	21.4	7.0	3.0
Indian	81.7	7.8	6.5	2.2
Pakistani	76.7	10.4	9.6	2.2
Bangladeshi	44.5	37.0	9.6	6.1

Source: 1991 Census

Bangladeshi households. Owner-occupation among Indians was highest (81.7 per cent), in contrast with Bangladeshis (44.5 per cent), as presented in Table 5.1.

The Pakistani households also show a higher owner-occupation rate (76.7 per cent) than the white households. However, renting from private landlords is higher among Pakistanis and Bangladeshis (both 9.6 per cent) than Indians (6.5 per cent) and whites (7 per cent). Renting from the public sector was highest among Bangladeshi households (37 per cent), compared with 10.4 per cent Pakistanis and only 7.8 per cent Indians. A survey in 1982 (Brown 1984) also revealed that the Asian housing owner-occupied rate was higher (72 per cent) than that of whites (59 per cent). However, it had also shown that, among Asians, Pakistanis in the sample had the highest owner-occupation rate (80 per cent), compared with Indians (77 per cent) and Bangladeshis with the lowest (30 per cent). The majority of Bangladeshis were renting from local councils (53 per cent) or from private landlords (11 per cent), but few Indians and Pakistanis were in this situation. It is worth mentioning that a large number of Sikh households in the sample (91 per cent) were owner-occupiers and few (6 per cent) were council tenants. It appears that these trends are continuing among young Asians.

The more recent PSI Survey (Modood *et al.* 1997) also confirmed the high levels of home ownership for Asians, except Bangladeshis. It showed that 85 per cent of Indians, 84 per cent of African Asians and 79 per cent of Pakistanis in the sample were owner-occupiers, compared with 48 per cent of Bangladeshis, as shown in Table 5.2.

The figures from the PSI Survey of 1982 in Table 5.2 show how the owner-occupation rate among different ethnic groups had changed in the twelve-year period. It is worth pointing out that,

Table 5.2 Housing tenure by ethnic group, 1982 and 1994 (percentages)

Housing tenure	White	Caribbean	Indian	African Asian	Pakistani	Bangla-deshi
1982 survey						
Owner-occupier	60	40	76	75	80	30
Social tenant	31	55	19	19	13	58
Private tenant	9	4	5	6	6	13
1994 survey						
Owner-occupier	67	50	85	84	79	48
Social tenant	23	46	9	12	15	45
Private tenant	9	4	7	5	6	8
Change 1982–94						
Owner-occupier	+7	+10	+9	+9	−1	+18
Social tenant	−8	−9	−10	−7	+2	−13
Private tenant	0	0	+2	−1	0	−5

Source: PSI/SCPR 1994 Survey (Modood *et al.* 1997); PSI 1982 Survey (Brown 1984)

while the owner-occupation rate for all ethnic groups has improved, it did not change significantly for Pakistanis. It appears that the improvement is partly due to the introduction of the Conservative government's policies in the 1980s when local authority tenants were given encouragement to buy their houses from their local councils. This policy has, it appears, also helped the owner-occupation of Bangladeshis, since the majority of them lived in local authority accommodation.

In our survey of 1983, we also found that 77 per cent of Asian young people were living in owner-occupied houses, compared with 46 per cent of white young people. One reason for this difference, compared with the patterns for whites mentioned above, seems to be that while 80 per cent of Asian young people lived with their parents, this was the case for only 69 per cent of white young people.

In our survey, we asked respondents whether they were satisfied with their housing conditions. The vast majority of Asian parents and young people (both 81 per cent) were satisfied. However, those who were not satisfied said that the condition of the house was bad and that they could not get repairs done. They also mentioned needing a bigger house, a consequence of the bigger size of Asian households. We found that the average household size for young Asians in the survey was 5.1 persons, compared with 3.9 persons for whites in the sample, while the national average for whites shown in the 1981 Census was 2.7 persons. The reason that our white sample had bigger households was simply because young people in the survey were from households with children of a particular age, and this excluded households without children or households with small children. However, this pattern could be checked by using the 1991 Census data.

The 1991 Census showed that the size of Asian households (4.2) was almost double that of white households (2.4). However, there were differences between various Asian groups: Indian (3.8), Pakistani (4.8) and Bangladeshi (5.3). This means that among Asians, Indian households are the smallest and Bangladeshi the largest. As pointed out in Chapter 2, Bangladeshi households have a larger number of dependent children aged up to 18 (3.4), compared to an average of 2.5 dependent children for all Asian households (OPCS 1993). At the other end of the scale, white households have a lot more elderly people than those of Asians. For example, the 1991 Census revealed that, while over a quarter (25.7 per cent) of white households were pensioner households, this was only the case for 2.8 per cent of Asian households. Among Asians, the Indians have a higher percentage of pensioner-headed households (3.6 per cent), the Bangladeshis the lowest (1.0 per cent), and Pakistanis (1.4 per cent).

Many Asians solve the housing problem by getting poor quality housing. This leads to disadvantages in terms of lack of amenities, overcrowding and concentration in neighbourhoods. One striking difference between whites and Asians is that among the whites owner-occupation is most common among the higher socio-economic groups, while council housing is most common among the lower socio-economic groups. For example, in 1974, a national survey revealed that 85 per cent of Asian households in the unskilled manual group were owner-occupiers, compared with only 20 per cent of white households in the same group (Smith 1976). A similar pattern was discovered in another national survey in 1982, which showed that 72 per cent of unskilled manual Asian heads of households were owner-occupiers compared with only 21 per cent of white heads of households in the same group (Brown 1984). This was despite Margaret Thatcher's government's emphasis on increasing home ownership among all sections of the population. However, higher ownership among unskilled Asians with low incomes means that they are often less able to maintain and improve their houses, which leads to further problems. When we examine the age of properties occupied by Asians and whites, clear differences emerge. For example, 26 per cent of Asian households were living in property built after 1945, compared with 50 per cent of white households. Therefore, the condition of many Asian households was determined not only by their incomes but also by the type and age of the property.

The higher owner-occupation rate among Asians, for example, could be deceptive in relation to their incomes and higher achievement in the housing market. This can be examined by looking at the type and quality of housing occupied by Asians compared with white people. Some research on the types of house owned by Asians and other ethnic minorities shows that the poor quality of many houses makes them become a liability rather than a satisfaction (Karn *et al.* 1985). More recent information about the types of house occupied by Asians was revealed by the PSI 1994 Survey referred to above (Modood *et al.* 1997). The survey showed that over half of the whites, Indians and African Asians were living in detached or semi-detached houses, compared with only 28 per cent of Pakistanis and 20 per cent of Bangladeshis. See Table 5.3 for details.

It is clear from Table 5.3 that almost two-thirds of Pakistanis and 42 per cent of Bangladeshis lived in terraced houses, while 37

Table 5.3 Types of accommodation: Asian groups and whites, 1982 and 1994 (percentages)

Type of accommodation	White	Indian	African Asian	Pakistani	Bangladeshi
1982 survey					
Detached/semi-	54	30	38	13	9
Terraced	31	57	48	80	39
Flat/other	15	13	13	7	52
1994 survey					
Detached/semi-	56	55	55	28	20
Terraced	27	33	31	64	42
Flat/other	16	13	13	7	37
Change 1982–94					
Detached/semi-	+2	+25	+17	+15	+11
Terraced	−4	−24	−17	−16	+3
Flat/other	+1	0	0	0	−15

Source: Adapted from the PSI/SCPR 1994 Survey (Modood *et al.* 1997); PSI 1982 Survey (Brown 1984)

per cent of Bangladeshis lived in flats and other types of accommodation. One of the explanations for the differences between Indians and African Asians in having more detached or semi-detached houses than Pakistanis and Bangladeshis seems to be that, generally, the latter groups live in inner-city areas, whereas a significant number of Indians and African Asians tend to live in outer-city areas. Table 5.3 also gives comparable figures from the PSI 1982 Survey. It shows that, overall, an improvement has taken place in 1994 for all Asian groups, compared with 1982 when fewer of them occupied detached or semi-detached houses.

Do Asians have enough accommodation in relation to their needs? The Bangladeshis had small accommodation compared to their needs and were sharing their dwellings most frequently. Sixty per cent of Bangladeshi families had more than one person per room, compared with only 3 per cent of whites, 26 per cent of Indians and 47 per cent of Pakistanis (Brown 1984). This pattern of overcrowding among Asians, particularly Bangladeshis, was confirmed by the 1991 Census, although there appears to be some improvement in this respect. In 1991, nearly half (47.1 per cent) of Bangladeshi families had more than one person per room, compared with 12.8 per cent of Indian, 29.7 per cent of Pakistani and only 1.8 per cent of white households in this situation. One explanation for this difference is the larger households of Bangladeshis and Pakistanis and the non-availability of big enough houses. This brings us to the basic amenities available to these households.

There appears to be considerable improvement in terms of the basic amenities in the last twenty years. This applies to Asians as well. In 1974, it was found that 37 per cent of Asian and West Indian households lacked the exclusive use of hot water or an inside WC, compared with 18 per cent white households. However, in 1982, there were only 7 per cent of Asian and West Indian households compared with 5 per cent of white households without basic amenities (Brown 1984). More recently, the 1991 Census revealed that there was little difference between the percentages of white households (1.2 per cent) and Asian households (1.4 per cent) which share a bathroom or WC. Among Asians, Bangladeshis have the highest percentage (2 per cent), Indians the lowest (1.1 per cent) of households without the exclusive use of these amenities; Pakistanis are midway (1.7 per cent). It appears from the evidence, as a whole, on housing conditions that the Bangladeshis have the worst housing conditions, not only among the Asian groups but also compared with the general population. There are several explanations for this. The first is that they are more recent arrivals; particularly, their dependents have arrived in the last few years. The second is that a majority of them live in rented accommodation, which is normally in a bad state of repair. Thirdly, they are heavily concentrated in the East End of London, where local authority districts have one of the highest levels of social and material deprivation. For example, Tower Hamlets, where Bangladeshis constitute 22.9 per cent of the total population, was ranked the fifth highest district in England in terms of social deprivation and the eighth highest in terms of material deprivation. Then, over a third of Bangladeshis are unemployed, and those in work are mainly in semi-skilled occupations which have lower wages. All these factors cause Bangladeshis to live in the worst housing conditions.

Information from the General Household Survey (GHS) also confirms the trend towards density of occupation, i.e. number of persons per room and the number of bedrooms in relation to the bedroom standard (Breeze *et al.* 1991). The GHS showed that 43 per cent of Pakistani and Bangladeshi, 22 per cent of Indian but only 6 per cent of white households had over one person per room. The survey also found only 2 per cent of white households with one or more bedrooms below the standard, compared with 13 per cent of Indian and 28 per cent of Pakistani and Bangladeshi households in this situation.

Some have argued that comparisons at national level of housing quality between whites and ethnic minorities could be misleading and that local-level comparison in this context would be more appropriate (Jones 1993). Therefore, we use one local area, Birmingham, for the analysis to see whether the patterns are any different to those reported above.

A survey in the 1970s in the Birmingham Handsworth area found that 81.6 per cent of Asians in the sample were owner-occupiers, compared to 41.25 per cent of whites (Rex and Tomlinson 1979). In 1982, it was found that 76 per cent of Asian households were owner-occupied in the West Midlands Metropolitan County, compared to 47 per cent of white households. On the other hand, 41 per cent of whites in the area were renting from the council, compared with only 19 per cent Asians (Brown 1984). The 1981 Census revealed a similar tenure pattern. It showed that 68

per cent of all New Commonwealth and Pakistani-origin households were owner-occupied, compared with 52 per cent of all
households in owner-occupation in Birmingham.

The 1991 Census provides us with the latest information about
housing tenure and housing amenities in Birmingham. It shows
that owner-occupation amongst Pakistanis is higher than amongst
white households. For example, 77.7 per cent of Pakistani and 84.6
per cent of Indian households were owner-occupied, compared to
60.7 per cent owner-occupation for white households in Birmingham (see Table 5.4). On the other hand, 27.7 per cent of Birmingham's white and 23.2 per cent of Bangladeshi households live in
local authority accommodation, while only 10.7 per cent of Pakistani households are in council housing.

Table 5.4 Tenure and ethnic group of household head, Birmingham, 1991
(percentages)

Ethnic group	Owner-occupied	Rented from LA	Rented privately	Rented from housing association
Indian	84.6	6.7	5.3	3.4
White	60.7	27.7	6.5	5.1
Pakistani	77.7	10.7	8.9	2.6
Bangladeshi	57.8	23.2	12.2	6.8
Black Caribbean	44.6	34.2	5.7	15.4

Source: 1991 Census

This tenure pattern in Birmingham for Pakistanis and Indians does
not explain their housing conditions. A higher proportion of Pakistani and Bangladeshi households than white ones in Birmingham
lack basic amenities. One in three Pakistani and more than 40 per
cent of Bangladeshi households, according to the 1991 Census,
were categorised as being overcrowded (more than one person per
room), compared with only 2 per cent of white households, as
presented in Table 5.5.

Table 5.5 also shows housing amenities and the availability of
central heating by ethnic group. If we compare the information in
Tables 5.4 and 5.5 with the national picture regarding Asians, the
pattern of ethnic differences between whites and Asians does not
change in any significant way.

In our survey of young Asian people, we asked respondents
whether they were satisfied with their housing conditions. Asians

Table 5.5 Household size, amenities, overcrowding and central heating
by ethnic group, Birmingham, 1991 (percentages)

Ethnic group	Average household size	Overcrowding: 1 + person per room	Lack of basic amenities	No central heating
Indian	4.3	16.1	1.0	29.9
White	2.3	2.0	1.5	36.8
Pakistani	5.2	32.7	1.9	62.4
Bangladeshi	5.7	42.0	1.5	55.9
Black Caribbean	2.5	4.1	1.0	32.5

Source: 1991 Census

generally and Bangladeshis in particular were less likely to be satisfied with their housing conditions than whites. Forty-three per cent of all Asian young people claimed to be very satisfied with their housing conditions, compared to 56 per cent of white young people, but only 12 per cent Bangladeshis made this claim. At the other end of the scale, 22 per cent of Bangladeshi young people were dissatisfied with their housing conditions, compared with 13 per cent whites. Lack of space, poor decorative state and dampness were the main reasons given by Asians and white people, although more Asians complained about the lack of space because of their bigger households. Relatively more Asians mentioned needing a bigger house.

One of the reasons that Asians live in concentrations is because of Asian shops and other community facilities. In both our 1975 and 1983 surveys, a majority of them said that they enjoyed living in an area where there were other Asian families. More Asian parents expressed this view than young Asians. They also mentioned the good community spirit and being near to people of their own race and culture as advantages. The first generation Asians, more so than the second, live in a close community. The main reason appears to be community facilities – shops, mosques, temples, etc., easier communication, friends around when in trouble or for advice. One respondent explained, 'we understand each other's way of living and feel at home'. However, apart from the cultural reasons for Asian concentrations, a significant number of Asians believed that they live together as a result of the hostility towards Asians shown by some sections of the white population. They also believed that racial prejudice and discrimination militates against Asians getting housing in 'good areas'. In our 1975 survey, over 45 per cent of Asian parents and young people expressed this view. One respondent explained:

> we do not get good houses. They do not even let us look at good houses. I have faced discrimination personally. In better areas such as this in which I am living, it was refused for me by the estate agent, solicitor, but I tried hard to get it.

Similar views and experiences were mentioned in our 1983 survey of Asians.

RACIAL DISCRIMINATION IN HOUSING

Racial discrimination in housing takes the form of white people being housed by local authorities in preference to Asians and those of other ethnic minorities, or of discriminatory attitudes and behaviour by landlords, estate agents and/or accommodation agencies. The CRE's formal investigation into council housing in the London Borough of Hackney and Tower Hamlets and its research and a formal investigation in Liverpool, referred to above, showed widespread discrimination against ethnic minority applicants and tenants. In private sector housing, discrimination, though undeclared, is still taking place, and this includes estate agents, private landlords and even building societies (CRE 1985c, 1990). Housing segregation has clear implications for education, and also bad housing will no doubt affect physical and mental health.

The evidence from our 1983 survey showed that a small proportion of the Asian respondents claimed that they were given the worst areas. Five per cent of Asian parents and 6 per cent of young Asians had experienced personal discrimination in housing. This had taken the form of being refused accommodation because of colour, having to wait for a long time for a good house, and being given the worst housing. Three comments are quoted to illustrate these points:

> We wanted to buy the house next door, they were white people. We asked them for a private deal which saves money. They said no and sold it through estate agents. If we were white they would have given us a deal.

> (Young Asian)

The white people get first choice and we are put at the bottom of the list and dumped.

(Mixed race young person)

Ethnic people get flats. They only get flats not houses with gardens. It takes longer to get a flat. There is no proper publicity for rent rebates. They should have these, translated, into Bengali particularly.

(Asian parent)

We asked young people and their parents for their views on the extent of racial discrimination in housing. Twenty-one per cent of young Asians and 16 per cent of Asian parents said that a great deal or quite a lot of racial discrimination existed in housing. It is interesting to point out that 29 per cent of white young people and 33 per cent of white parents also thought that there was a great deal or quite a lot of discrimination in housing. The examples of the nature of this discrimination mentioned included: white people get better houses, whites have less trouble in renting, and whites do not like people from ethnic minorities living next door. If this is how some Asians feel about their position in housing, are policy makers aware of their concerns and experience, and what relevant action are they are taking to deal with these?

We interviewed forty-four councillors as part of our survey in areas where there were large numbers from ethnic minorities. The councillors were asked, in particular, about the housing needs of young people. Fifty-nine per cent of the councillors thought that lack of accommodation was a problem facing all young people. However, 25 per cent of the councillors felt that Asians and other ethnic minority young people did have different housing needs. The main differences perceived by these councillors were that ethnic minorities tended to have larger families and therefore needed larger houses. One councillor said:

There is a need for four- to five-bedroomed houses and for much larger sums of money for repairs and improvement. They [ethnic minorities] are living in poorer housing, generally.

Also, ethnic minorities generally, and Asians in particular, were seen to have different housing needs to the white population because there was assumed to be more intergenerational conflict and more need for Asian young people to have their own accommodation. One councillor explained this belief:

The generation gap is much greater – individuals are more likely to be thrown out of the family home, and so need housing . . . we are now monitoring the position carefully. Accusations have been that not enough has been done so we have decided to encourage housing associations to provide single-person flats.

The councillors were also asked whether the council had taken any action to cater specifically for the housing needs of Asians and other ethnic minorities. Most of them said that no such action had been taken, several commenting that everybody was treated the same and rehousing was purely on the basis of need. However, some councillors mentioned special provision and one gave an example:

Improvement grants have been given to try to improve the housing in areas which Asians have chosen to live, where property is often older and back to back.

Another councillor mentioned the need for special provision for young people.

We are certainly looking to furnish accommodation for students and young, single people – a high proportion of black young men with a generation gap problem with parents.

Finally, councillors were asked whether their council had any plans to implement any new policies with regard to the housing needs of ethnic minority young people. Most councillors said they knew of no such policy or that they would just continue existing policy. One councillor said that his local authority was encouraging housing associations to provide single-person flats, while another mentioned proposals for special hostels for young persons in general, which would also benefit Asian young people.

Compared with the experience of Asian young people in education and employment, their experience in housing is not too bad. Although they have some concerns about the quality of housing and racial discrimination in housing allocations and the housing market, their contact with this market is limited. Bangladeshis, in particular, face acute problems in housing allocations and in terms of housing conditions because they are in the rented housing market, compared with Indians and Pakistanis, the overwhelming majority of whom are in owner-occupied accommodation. They also face some disadvantages, as mentioned above, but because they are owner-occupiers their day-to-day contact with the housing market is relatively limited.

Chapter 6

Racial harassment and race relations

In the 1980s and, more recently, in 1995 and 1996 there was unprecedented violence in some inner-city areas of Britain. The frustrations of young people generally and young Asians and young Afro-Caribbeans in particular became apparent during these disturbances. The present economic situation has not helped in this context. Anxieties and feelings of insecurity among Asian young people have recently increased. Too many young Asians feel frustrated and see no future for themselves. They also see an increasing number of racial attacks and racial harassment incidents, particularly against Asians.

[handwritten: → compare with Recent Bradius study]

RACIAL ATTACKS AND HARASSMENT

One Home Office study showed that in 1981 the rate of racial attacks against Asians was fifty times that for white people (Home Office 1981). This was confirmed by the Select Committee Report on this subject published in 1986 (Home Affairs Committee 1986). Another report by the Home Office in 1989 highlighted once again the phenomenon of racial attacks and harassment (Home Office 1989). The most common form of racial attack was by whites against Asians, who comprised 70 per cent of the victims of recorded incidents in London. The victim was usually a woman or child, the attacker a white teenager, often part of a gang, and sometimes encouraged by white parents. Figures from the Metropolitan Police show that the number of racial attacks recorded has increased generally and against Asians in particular in the recent past. Several serious cases against Asians, particularly against Bangladeshis, in the East End of London received wide publicity in the media and also resulted in public demonstrations against this sort of violence against Asians. In this context there are also an increasing number of racial harassment cases and racial attacks which take place on some local authority housing estates (CRE 1987b). This was confirmed by the Home Affairs Committee Report (1989 and 1994) on racial attacks and harassment, which made appropriate recommendations to local authorities and to the police to take such incidents seriously and asked them to tackle these as one of their priority tasks. The Home Office also published a report entitled *The Response to Racial Attacks and Harassment* (1989) showing the urgency of action in this field.

The Home Affairs Committee, in its report in the mid-1980s on *Racial Attacks and Harassment*, said 'the most shameful and dispiriting aspects of race relations in Britain is the incidence of racial attacks and harassment' (Home Affairs Committee 1986). In 1989, the Home Affairs Committee looked at these issues again and concluded that there was a significant level of under-reporting of racial incidents. In 1994, it was reported that there were about 130,000 incidents of crime and threats against Asian and Afro-Caribbean people (*Guardian*, 11 February 1994). Therefore, the police figures of only a few thousand racially motivated crimes per year nationally are nowhere near the reality, because many people do not report such incidents and because they know that the police have a poor detection rate for such incidents. For example, in London in 1989 the clear-up rate for racial incidents was just over 30 per cent. However, as a result of increased publicity of such incidents, more ethnic minority people are coming forward to report racial incidents. Two further points are worth making: (1) that racial attacks on individuals affect not just one person but whole families and their friends, and (2) that it is estimated that, between 1970 and 1989, 74 people died as a result of racially motivated attacks (Gordon 1990).

In 1990, the then Metropolitan Police Commissioner, Sir Peter Imbert, wrote 'racial attacks are not only against the law, they are also socially divisive and morally repugnant'. The Home Affairs Committee added to this:

> we would go further. We believe that if racism is allowed to grow unchecked it will begin to corrode the fabric of our open and tolerant society. For this reason crimes and anti-social behaviour become more serious when they are racially motivated than when they are not. This belief lies at the core of our

review of this subject and our recommendations.

(Home Affairs Committee 1994)

The fact that the Home Affairs Committee published three reports within eight years on racial attacks and harassment (1986, 1989 and 1994) shows the serious nature of the subject and its likely impact on race relations.

The British Crime Survey in 1991 showed that 56 per cent of racially motivated incidents involving Asians were assaults and 66 per cent were seen as threats (Home Office 1992). However, racial violence in any form creates a climate of fear, intimidation and insecurity. One development is that there is now a greater recognition of this problem at government levels. For example, the Home Secretary, speaking at the Conservative Party Con- ference in October 1993, said, 'racial attacks will not be tolerated, and those who perpetrate them must be caught, convicted and punished'. It is clear, however, from officially recorded figures that the number of reported racial incidents is increasing every year. For example, in 1989, the cases reported to the police in Britain were 5,420 and this number increased to over 10,000 in 1994 (see Table 6.1 for details).

Table 6.1   Reported racial incidents in Britain, 1989–94

Police area	1989	1990	1991	1992	1993	1994*
Provincial police total	2,347	3,451	4,509	4,566	5,329	5,873
Metropolitan police total	2,697	2,908	3,373	3,227	3,889	3,889[†]
England and Wales (including London)	5,044	6,359	7,882	7,793	9,218	9,762
Scotland	376	636	678	663	726	—
Total	5,420	6,995	8,560	8,456	9,944	—

Source: Home Office figures, quoted in Skellington 1996
* April 1993 to January 1994.
[†] Police estimate.

This means that reported racial incidents almost doubled within the five-year period. However, we know that this number only represents the tip of the iceberg (Virdee 1995). Also, 'low'-level racially motivated incidents are recorded neither by the police nor by the British Crime Survey, referred to above, which estimated racially motivated crimes to be 130,000 every year. Recently, a minister at the Home Office estimated them to be 140,000 a year.

However, the Labour Party estimated them at between 175,000 and 200,000 a year (Ruddock 1994), which is higher than other recent estimates.

Several studies have shown that racial attacks affect Asians more than some other ethnic groups (Mayhew *et al.* 1989). The CRE revealed in 1993 that 49 per cent of victims of racial attacks were Asian, 23 per cent Afro-Caribbean, 22 per cent white and 7 per cent Jewish (CRE 1993). Asian shopkeepers and Asian women seem to be special targets of racial attacks. For example, one study in London in 1993 showed that 32 per cent of Asian shopkeepers were racially abused within one twelve-month period, and this figure rose to 37 per cent in the Midlands (Hibberd and Shapland 1993). This seems to be the pattern in other areas of Asian settlement. Asian women have recently become targets and had their jewellery and purses snatched. Such incidents have resulted in serious injuries to many Asian women and created a feeling of intimidation and insecurity among Asians.

In our 1983 survey, young Asians and parents were asked how serious they considered racial attacks in their area to be. It showed that more young Asians (38 per cent) than parents (29 per cent) saw racial attacks as very or fairly serious. Details are presented in Table 6.2.

Table 6.2 Extent to which racial attacks are a problem

Seen as	Asian young people %	Asian parents %
Very/fairly serious	38	28
Not very/not at all serious	55	55
Don't know	7	5
Size of sample	570	212

It is worth noting that relatively more Asian parents did not know. Many interviews with young people in 1993/4 also confirmed that young Asians were more aware of the issue of racial harassment than their parents were. This is partly explained by their more frequent contact with white people, but also due to their personal experience in educational institutions and employment.

When asked whether they, or any of their family or friends, had ever been physically attacked by someone of a different racial group, and, if so, whether they felt the attack was racially motivated, 34 per cent of Asian young people and 21 per cent of Asian parents said that either they themselves, or a family member or a friend, had been attacked, as presented in Table 6.3. Over 70 per cent of young Asians claimed that these attacks were racially motivated.

Table 6.3 Experience of racial attacks

Experience	Asian young people %	Asian parents %
No one attacked	71	76
Attacked		
Self	11	5
Family	11	8
Friend	12	8
Size of sample	570	212

Table 6.3 confirms the greater awareness and experience of young Asians regarding racial attacks. It is worth pointing out that some of the racial attacks are organised by racist organisations or show racial hostility; some attacks are unprovoked, where no racial motive is stated; and another type, relevant here, is theft or attempted theft. The incidence of such attacks is higher in major conurbations and higher still in the inner-city areas of these conurbations where the majority of the Asians live.

What were the attitudes of Asians towards racial attacks and racial insults? A survey in 1982 (Brown 1984) asked: 'Would you say physical attacks for racial reasons and/or racialist insults directed at people of Asian/West Indian origin have got better than they were five years ago, about the same, or got worse?' The answers are reproduced in Table 6.4. The table also provides an interesting gender dimension. Generally the majority of both Asian men and women felt that the situation had become worse, with few believing it had improved.

It is clear that Asian men show greater awareness of the situation, and almost 30 per cent of Asian women did not express an opinion. As mentioned above, a more recent Home Office study showed that there were 130,000 racially motivated criminal incidents recorded every year. Of these, 32,500 were assaults, 52,000 were threats and 26,000 involved vandalism. It also showed that one in five Asians living in inner-city areas felt that racial attacks

Table 6.4 Racial attacks and racial insults: beliefs and
trends (percentages)

Opinion	Asian men	Asian women
Physical attacks		
Better	6	4
Same	22	17
Worse	52	50
Don't know	20	28
Racialist insults		
Better	5	3
Same	24	19
Worse	54	50
Don't know	17	28

Source: Adapted from Brown 1984

were a 'very big' or 'fairly big' problem (*Guardian*, 11 February
1994). It is, however, worth pointing out that many victims of
racial harassment and racial attacks do not report them to the
police and, therefore, the true picture is never revealed in the
official statistics. Some Asians claimed that they do not report
such incidents because they know the police would not take any
action. One respondent explained this to the author in 1994 in the
following way:

> I know from my personal experience and from the experience of
> some other Asians in Birmingham that reporting racial harass-
> ment and racial attacks cases to the police is a wastage of time.
> Also, if you report the police in turn start asking awkward
> questions and sometimes make us feel as if we, as Asians, are
> criminals and not victims of racism.

(Asian young person)

This attitude and experience show that there is a lack of trust
between some sections of the Asian population and the police. In
our survey, Asians and Asian parents were asked to rate police
protection against racial attacks in their area. Two-thirds of Asian
young people and 58 per cent of Asian parents thought that the level
of police protection was average to poor, as shown in Table 6.5.

It is worth noting that one in five parents could not give an
opinion of police protection and, once again, more young Asians
thought police protection was poor. Young Asians were asked

Table 6.5 Comparison of young Asians' and Asian parents' opinion of police protection

Opinion	Young people %	Parents %
Good	15	20
Average	42	43
Poor	24	15
Don't know	12	21
Size of sample	570	212

Source: 1983 survey

whether they had ever been stopped and searched by the police and or had a brush with the law. Eighteen per cent of young Asians claimed to have been stopped and searched and harassed by the police. Six per cent of the respondents appeared in courts as defendant and 2 per cent were sentenced in court. It is worth pointing out that the Afro-Caribbean young people interviewed at the same time were more likely than Asians and whites to say that they had been stopped and searched (39 per cent) or been harassed by the police (27 per cent), had appeared in court as a defendant (26 per cent) and sentenced in court (13 per cent). The main forms of harassment by police mentioned by Asian and Afro-Caribbean young people were: stopping and searching without reason, verbal threats, and physical violence or pushing. One extreme example of harassment was mentioned by an Asian young person:

> I was stopped on the street for carrying three cricket stumps. After investigation, I was allowed to go but was advised to carry them in a bag in future.

The street disturbances in Bradford in June 1995 also showed that there was still a great deal of mistrust between young Asians and the police in the area. In fact, the whole trouble started when a policeman started questioning a few young Asians who claimed that they were playing football. It appears, generally, that in some areas police community relations are not very good. In this context, we can present some findings from our survey of Asian parents who were asked to rate the relation between the police and the local community on a scale ranging from very good (5) through to very bad (1). Table 6.6 shows the opinions.

It is clear that just over half of the respondents felt that relations between the police and local community were either good or very

Table 6.6 Asian parents' opinion of relations between police and local community

Opinion	%
(Very) good	52
Neither good nor bad	24
(Very) bad	9
Don't know	14
Mean score	3.5
Size of sample	212

Source: 1983 survey

good, but almost a third said that either they were bad or very bad or neither good nor bad, and 14 per cent did not express view. These opinions certainly raise questions about the effectiveness of community policing, and the efforts which have been made by the Home Office and some police forces towards the training of police officers to police multi-racial areas of Britain.

Attitudes and beliefs are as important as facts. Therefore, we had also asked our respondents in another survey (Anwar 1981) some questions about their perceptions of relations between the police and ethnic minorities and whether these relations were better or worse than for white people. Only 5 per cent of the 330 Asian respondents thought ethnic minorities had better relations, 43 per cent thought they had worse relations and 33 per cent agreed that the relations were the same. However, when these responses were analysed with age, 61 per cent of ethnic minority young people (including Asians) said that they had worse relations with the police than the white community. This survey also confirmed perceptions that the relations between the police and ethnic minorities were not very good.

The PSI Survey 1994 also asked for views on a statement about police protection from racial harassment, namely, 'Black and Asian people can rely on the police to protect them from racial harassment.' The results show that only a third of Asian respondents agreed with this statement and relatively more young Asians disagreed, as presented in Table 6.7.

The results show that the Asian young in particular were not optimistic about police protection.

Respondents were also asked if black and Asian people should organise self-defence groups to protect themselves from racial

Table 6.7 'Black and Asian people can rely on the police to protect them' (percentages)

Response	All South Asian respondents	16–34-year-old South Asian respondents
Agree/agree strongly	35	33
Neither agree nor disagree	13	11
Disagree/disagree strongly	43	50
Can't say	9	6

Source: Adapted from SCPR/PSI Survey 1994 (Modood *et al*. 1997)

Table 6.8 Self-defence groups to protect themselves (percentages)

Response	Caribbeans	Asians
Agree/agree strongly	49	52
Neither agree nor disagree	11	14
Disagree/disagree strongly	31	24
Can't say	9	9

Source: SCPR/PSI Survey 1994 (Modood *et al*. 1997)

attacks. The majority of Asians agreed with this, as shown in Table 6.8.

The results seems to be consistent with the view, held by many young Asians in particular, that if the police are failing to protect Asians, then they should organise self-defence groups to protect themselves. One young Asian girl explained:

> Asians generally, but Asian women in particular, are seen by some whites and some West Indians as soft and easy target because they wear a lot of jewellery and are unable to defend themselves. In our area, the police have failed to stop such incidents and I think the community should get organised to defend their women.
>
> (Interview 1994)

In fact, in some areas of Asian settlements some Asian vigilante groups were organised, in particular in the East End of London.

It is relevant to mention here that a significant number of Asians reported some form of racial harassment in the previous twelve months, as shown in Table 6.9.

The survey showed that, within Asian groups, a higher proportion of African Asians and Pakistanis reported being subjected to

Table 6.9 Racial harassment in the previous twelve months, by gender and ethnic group (percentages)

Ethnic group	Male	Female	Total
Indian	12	8	10
African Asian	16	10	14
Pakistani	15	11	13
Bangladeshi	10	7	9

Source: SCPR/PSI Survey 1994 (Modood *et al.* 1997)

some form of racial harassment than of Indians and Bangladeshis. It is worth pointing out that 4 per cent of Pakistani, 3 per cent of Bangladeshi, 2 per cent of Indian and 2 per cent of African Asian respondents said that they had been physically attacked in the previous twelve months. The survey also found that 13 per cent of Indians, African Asians and Pakistanis and 7 per cent of Bangladeshis reported damage done to their property in the last twelve months because of their race or colour. However, about half of those respondents who had reported racial harassment to the police were dissatisfied with the police response (Modood *et al.* 1997). On the whole, it appears that racial harassment and racial attacks against Asians, but also against other ethnic groups, are a serious problem and that people worry about being racially attacked. For example, the 1994 survey referred to above showed that 32 per cent of African Asians and 22 per cent of Indians, Pakistanis and Bangladeshis worry about being racially harassed. This sort of situation certainly affects attitudes towards race relations. Lord Scarman stressed in 1981, when he was carrying out his inquiry into the Brixton disorders, that 'The point has often been put to this Inquiry, and I think everybody accepts it, that we are as much concerned with attitudes and beliefs as we are with facts.' Many surveys during the period since have used questions on 'race relations', but I have selected only a few to show the trends over time.

RACE RELATIONS

In a survey in 1975 (Kohler 1976), it was revealed that 43 per cent of Asians felt that race relations were getting better and only 11 per cent thought that race relations were getting worse in the country as a whole, and 33 per cent of Asians said that race relations were

remaining the same. Those questions were repeated in a follow-up
survey in 1981 (Anwar 1981). This survey showed a dramatically
different picture from that revealed in the 1975 survey. In the 1981
survey more than four out of ten (43 per cent) of the Asian
respondents thought that race relations were getting worse and
only 16 per cent thought they were getting better, while the figure
for those who said race relations remained the same was no different (33 per cent) to that in 1975. It is interesting to note from the
1981 survey that among the Asians, those born in Britain and those
more fluent in English were more likely to think race relations had
deteriorated. Another survey (Brown 1984), which used a different
wording for questions, gave us further details about Asians' views
on life in Britain, but it also showed differences between various
Asian groups. It indicated that only 15 per cent of Asians in the
sample thought that, in general, life in Britain was now better for
people of Asian/West Indian origin than it had been five years
earlier. Details are presented in Table 6.10.

Table 6.10 'Life in Britain improved for our ethnic group': Asian sample,
1974, and 1982 comparison (percentages)

	Asian		Indian		Pakistani		Bangla-deshi		African Asian	
	1974	1982	1974	1982	1974	1982	1974	1982	1974	1982
Better	35	15	40	16	31	12	—	4	32	21
Worse	18	51	17	50	21	54	—	53	18	47
No change	32	17	31	17	36	17	—	16	31	18
Don't know	14	16	12	16	12	17	—	26	19	14

Source: Adapted from Brown 1984

It is clear that, when compared with a similar survey in 1974
(Smith 1976), things were perceived to be a lot worse in 1982. Over
half of the Asians, as a group, said that their life in Britain had got
worse, compared with only 18 per cent in 1974, and, similarly, for
those who thought things had got better the situation was quite
different to that in the 1974 survey. Those who said that life in
Britain for ethnic minorities was worse were asked for their reasons. Sixty-seven per cent of Asians mentioned the recession as a
general reason and 49 per cent mentioned racial disadvantage
and racial discrimination. The reasons for the worsening of their

position in relation to white people included racist organisations and racial attacks.

The 1983 survey of young people also showed that less than one in five young Asians said that race relations had improved over the previous year or two, while just over half (54 per cent) felt that race relations remained the same. Table 6.11 shows the details and also includes how young Asians in the sample saw race relations developing over the next five years.

Table 6.11 Young Asians' and Asian parents' opinion on race relations

	Race relations in own area over previous year or two		Race relations generally over next five years	
	Young Asians %	*Parents* %	*Young Asians* %	*Parents* %
Better	19	11	16	5
Same	54	51	34	30
Worse	1	11	29	22
Don't know	15	55	21	42
Size of sample	570	212	570	212

While one in five did not give an opinion, over one third of the other sample were not optimistic about improving race relations in the future, but felt that race relations would get worse. Only 16 per cent of all young Asians said that race relations would get better, with 34 per cent saying race relations would remain the same and 29 per cent saying that they would get worse over the next five years. The main reason for thinking that race relations had got worse over the previous year or two was that there had been racial attacks or disturbances, mentioned by 44 per cent of Asian young people. It is worth pointing out that this survey was undertaken after the urban disturbances in Brixton, Bristol and Liverpool. When asked about their thinking that race relations would worsen in the future, over 60 per cent of those Asian young people thinking race relations would get worse said that the unemployment situation was the main reason for this. Also, 13 per cent of this group of respondents mentioned racial attacks and riots in the area, followed by another 11 per cent who believed that there would always be prejudice. Two comments of young Asians from the 1983 survey and 1994 research in this context are relevant here to illustrate the situation:

White people do not like increasing Asian concentration. High unemployment rate puts blame on Asians. It would be better if Asians were spread out.

(Young Asian 1983)

Whatever we do to succeed in education and employment, we are blamed for the higher unemployment and lower standard of education. We are also blamed for the housing conditions in inner-city areas – although Asian people keep their areas clean for the fear of backlash from white people. Due to increasing numbers of racial attacks, many more Asians living outside are now moving into Asian areas. One Asian said: race relations cannot improve in this sort of situation where Asians do not feel safe.

(Young Asian 1994)

Table 6.11 also shows Asian parents' views on race relations. A high proportion of Asian parents were unsure about the future but very few felt that either the race relations in their area had improved (11 per cent) or they would improve in the next five years (5 per cent). Like young Asians, parents mostly thought that the unemployment situation would lead to worsening race relations in the future and mentioned racial attacks and riots as a further reason. One Asian parent commented:

A lot of people these days are unemployed and coloured people will be picked up if they are still in employment or run their own businesses.

Some Asian parents had given examples of attacks on Asian businesses which were racially motivated; others mentioned damage to Asians' cars as a result of jealousy by some white people. In my more recent research, I have discovered that, in areas like Birmingham, young Asians are very aware of the increasing number of racial harassment incidents and the extent of racial prejudice and discrimination, which are affecting race relations. However, on the whole it appears that concerning racial attacks, relations with the police and race relations, young Asians are not very optimistic and more action needs to be taken by relevant institutions to turn this pessimism into some optimism about their future as British citizens.

Let us now examine how attitudes have changed about racial prejudice in the last decade or so.

The British Social Attitudes Survey in 1984 showed that 90 per cent of the respondents felt that British society was racially prejudiced against its black and Asian members (Jowell *et al.* 1984). Forty-two per cent of the respondents thought racial prejudice would be worse in five years, time, and in fact a third of them classified themselves as racially prejudiced.

Similar trends were found in 1991 in another survey of attitudes, commissioned by the Runnymede Trust (Amin and Richardson 1992). It showed that two out of every three white people thought Britain was a very or fairly racist society, compared to 78 per cent of Afro-Caribbeans and 56 per cent of Asians. Almost 40 per cent (39 per cent) of whites, 42 per cent of Asians but a high 67 per cent of Afro-Caribbeans believed that employers discriminated against non-white workers. A similar pattern of attitudes emerged regarding the police (worse 48 per cent white; 75 per cent Afro-Caribbean; and 45 per cent Asian). This survey also showed that over 60 per cent of Afro-Caribbeans, 45 per cent of Asians and 31 per cent of whites thought that British laws against racial discrimination were not tough enough, with the implication that some action was needed in this context.

The 1992 British Social Attitudes (BSA) survey confirmed that the public still perceived Britain as a racially prejudiced society (Jowell *et al.* 1992). A Gallup survey for the American Jewish Committee (1993) revealed that 25 per cent of white British would object to living next to non-white people, 10 per cent wanted anti-discrimination laws to be abolished, and 45 per cent of the total sample thought that anti-Semitism was not a problem. The survey also showed that the 'most racist respondents' tended to be working-class, elderly and the least educated. It is also interesting to point out that over three-quarters of respondents felt that race relations in Britain were 'only fair' or 'poor', and over 40 per cent thought that anti-racist laws should be strengthened. Once again there is support for more action. The more recent evidence is worrying. An ICM survey in July 1995, in 52 randomly selected constituencies, revealed that two-thirds of the respondents admitted to being racist, and only one in ten said that people they knew were not racist. Also, over half of the respondents believed that there was racial discrimination in the labour market (*Daily Express*, 8 August 1995). Therefore, the recent evidence suggests that, instead of the attitudes of whites towards Asians and other ethnic minorities improving, the situation seems to be getting worse and requires more action in providing information to ordinary white people that Asians and other ethnic minorities are British and a majority of them are British born.

Chapter 7

The family and marriage

Asians in Britain want to keep their cultural identity, including religious practices, distinguishing patterns of family customs, and mother tongue. At the same time, they adapt to other aspects of Western culture, such as the language, the education system, employment patterns, and the civic life of society. They would like understanding and acceptance of their identities by the white population and its institutions. The situation of young Asians will be examined in this context. The information from the two surveys (1975 and 1983) referred to in previous chapters will be used to show what changes in attitudes took place in almost ten years. Some more recent qualitative information will be used from interviews with young people, conducted by the author in 1993 and 1994. The parents' attitudes are important about religio-cultural issues and, therefore, a comparison of their attitudes, wherever possible and relevant, will be made with the attitudes of young Asians.

THE FAMILY

The traditional family system in India, Bangladesh and Pakistan is the joint and extended family. The joint/extended family consists of a group, usually of three or more generations, with a complex set of mutual obligations. They usually pool their income, and expenditure is controlled centrally and made from a common purse. It includes affinal relations, created by marriage, as well as those of descent. Brothers share land, prosperity and other business, work together and live together, if possible. In some cases, where one or two members of the family are working in other geographical areas or are working abroad, which is often the case for Asians in Britain, they still maintain family obligations and hold together as a joint family. Another type of family which exists in the sub-continent consists of a 'stem family', where aged parents live with one of their sons and his wife and children, other sons having established their own households. The traditional joint household then, in practice, divides into separate entities, each contributing labour and finance, and participating in the traditional gift exchange and birth, marriage and death ceremonies. In Britain, there are some large joint families whose members establish separate households because, even if they want to live together, the houses are not big enough.

It is worth pointing out here that the joint/extended family plays an important role in the life of an Asian individual. Many important decisions are made jointly. The other normal structural rules for the Asian family are: patrilineal descent group, patrilocal residential rule, patriarchal authority and respect related to age and sex, and preferential marriage patterns which lead to extended networks in the wider sense.

Migration has certainly modified and changed the structure and probably some of the functions of Asian joint families in Britain. If the joint family means, in a very loose sense, a system by which relatives maintain a relationship of some intimacy with members of a nuclear family, then such Asian families do exist in the urban conditions of Britain. However, there are pressures for change along with the continuity of the spirit of the traditional family system. To determine what changes have taken place in the Asian communities, it is important to examine those factors which affect the lives of Asians in Britain.

As mentioned above, due to the nature of migration and immigration restrictions, Asian extended families in Britain are less common than in the countries of origin. In Britain, the households are usually of two generations. Grandparents were less frequently found in Britain in 1975 than currently. In our survey of 1975, out of 1,427 Asian households, 67 per cent were living as nuclear families and 33 per cent as extended families. More Hindus (37 per cent) were living in extended families than Sikhs (32 per cent) and Muslims (29 per cent). This was partly due to the type of migration which took place, in which East African Asians, the majority of those being Hindus, had migrated as families, compared with Pakistanis and Bangladeshi Muslims, who were still in the process of bringing their 'families' to Britain, and had very few grandparents as dependants. The Asian families may change over

time when more families have grandchildren. Some Asian households in Britain included unmarried brothers of the husband or
wife in the 1970s. In some cases, married brothers live together as a
joint family, living mostly in the same household. A national survey
in 1982 (Brown 1984) revealed that 21 per cent of Asian households
had more than one family unit, African Asians having the highest
(26 per cent) and Indians the lowest (18 per cent) among Asians.
This survey also showed that several households were joint or
extended. Even in the 1990s, in some cases, married brothers live
together as a joint family, living mostly in the same house. In other
cases, due to the lack of availability of large houses, brothers live in
separate houses but function as a joint family. The 1991 Census
also showed that Asian households were larger (4.2 persons) than
white households (2.4 persons). It showed too that Asian households not only had more children but also more adults, which gives
an indication of the pattern described above.

What are the attitudes of Asians to the joint/extended family?
These will also help us to determine what patterns of Asian families
could develop in the future. In the 1975 survey, we discovered that
an overwhelming majority of both Asian parents and young people
– eight out of ten – believed that Asians preferred to live in joint
families. It is interesting that in the 1983 survey, exactly the same
percentage (80 per cent) of both Asian young people and Asian
parents once again agreed with the statement, which was repeated
in this survey. We had expected a change in attitudes after about
ten years. Only 14 per cent of our respondents had disagreed with
the statement in 1975, which came down to only 6 per cent in 1983.
Variations in both the surveys between religious groups were marginal, as indeed were differences between men and women, different
age groups, those with varying lengths of residence in Britain and
those born in Britain.

There were two interesting reasons mentioned for the continued
preference for the extended family system: the traditional and the
pragmatic. Remarks about the traditional view included: 'traditionally, families live together', 'they stick together', 'so that people can
help each other' and 'members of families rely on each other'. The
pragmatic reasons mentioned include: love of parents and recognition of the duty of looking after them, particularly in old age.
Several respondents in my recent interviews with young Asians
have also expressed similar views. One typical view mentioned by
a young Asian was that:

Asian parents pay so much attention to their families and work difficult shifts and do hard work for their children. I feel strongly that we should continue as a family unit and look after our parents in their old age. This is what makes us different than white and West Indian people. We have strong family units.

(Interview 1993)

Two more recent sources of information, the 1991 Census and the 1994 Fourth National Survey of Ethnic Minorities (Modood *et al*. 1997), give us some details about the nature of Asian families and how they differ from other ethnic groups. The 1991 Census showed that about one-third of South Asians were living in a household containing a nuclear family but with other permanent residents as well. The Census showed that Asians were much more likely to live in households containing at least two family units – about 15 per cent did so compared to 3 per cent black and only 1.5 per cent white households (Murphy 1996). See Table 7.1 for details.

Table 7.1 Asian and white family types, 1991 (percentages)

Ethnic group	One family only	One family and mono (s)*	Two or more monos*	One person only	At least two families
White	79.5	5.1	3.0	11.0	1.5
Indian	66.5	14.3	1.5	2.5	15.2
Pakistani	67.3	14.5	1.3	1.9	15.1
Bangladeshi	73.8	12.4	2.2	1.4	10.2

Source: Adapted from Murphy 1996, based on 1 per cent of Individual Anonymised Records (SAR) from the 1991 Census
* A mono might be a divorced child, a widow, a widower, an elderly parent, or a non-relative.

The Individual Anonymised Records (SAR) analysis also showed that multi-family households were not necessarily three-generation households. Asians were more likely to have more distant relations living in their households than white people were. Among the Asian groups, Indians were more likely to have vertically extended three-generation households than were Pakistanis and Bangladeshis, whose households were more likely to be horizontally extended, having normally more brothers and sisters living with the head of the household. See Table 7.2 for details.

It is clear that 55 per cent of Pakistani and Bangladeshi and 41 per cent of Indian households with two or more family units had

Table 7.2 Relationship of heads of 'secondary' family units in two or more family households to the head of household, Asian and white, 1991 (percentages)

Ethnic group	Child/child-in-law	Parent/parent-in-law	Sib/sib-in-law	Other relations	Other
White	79.9	10.5	3.0	1.4	5.1
Indian	58.7	25.0	11.5	1.4	3.4
Pakistani/ Bangladeshi	44.2	27.4	19.5	4.4	4.4

Source: Adapted from Murphy 1996

parents/parents-in-law and other relations living with the head of the households, compared with only 20 per cent of white families in this situation. The analysis also showed that there were no class differences to this pattern, for both whites and Asians.

The 1994 survey (Modood *et al.* 1997) also showed that a lot more Asians had complex household structures than did white households. For example, more than four out of five Asian single adults lived with their parents, compared with 59 per cent whites, as shown in Table 7.3.

It is clear from Table 7.3 that, compared with whites, many Asian married couples lived with their parents, and that Asian households were also more likely to have ex-married individuals. All this shows that, despite difficulties with finding large enough houses, many Asians live in extended households and many more who do not live in the same household function as joint families. The main reasons for preferring to live in a nuclear family were privacy, independence and having a home of one's own. Some Asians see that the nuclear family would also be less crowded.

Table 7.3 Proportion of family units aged less than 60 living with their parents, Asian and white (percentages)

Ethnic group	White	Indian/ Asian African	Pakistani/Bangladeshi
Single, no children	59	82	87
Single parents	12	n.a.	n.a.
Married couples	2	21	22
Ex-married individuals	9	14	17

Source: Adapted from SCPR/PSI Survey 1994 (Modood *et al.* 1997)

In our survey of 1975 (Anwar 1976), we asked both Asian parents and young Asians about their experience of living in an extended family. More parents (75 per cent) than young people (57 per cent) felt that they enjoyed the extended family. My more recent research has confirmed this generational difference. Parents of all the Asian religious groups equally enjoyed the extended family, while among young people, more Muslims expressed this feeling than Hindus and Sikhs. The major reason for favouring the extended family was the fact that it was part of the traditional way of life and that it made for a happier family on which the individual member could depend in time of need. One female respondent explained in this way:

> We have always lived that way. I like everybody around me. I am now getting old and I will be looked after. If I was on my own that would be difficult. I like to live in a big family and provided the accommodation is sufficient, I can keep the privacy of my own family unit.

The 1975 survey had also shown that the extended family system would not persist in the same way in the future. For example, 57 per cent of young Asians agreed with the statement: 'When I have a house of my own, I would prefer to have my husband/wife and children living with me.' However, a substantial minority of young Asians still preferred to live in an extended family.

Some of the more recent research on Asian groups (Warrier 1994) also shows that Asians are committed to the traditional joint family in which power is hierarchically distributed according to age and sex. However, in practice, the process of decision making and domestic division of labour among Prajabti Hindus was affected by the number, age and marital status of the sons living with parents, and also by the financial contribution of each member to the household income. On the other hand, nuclear Asian families are more flexible in terms of decision making (Vatuk 1972; Warrier, 1994). Wives in nuclear families usually take part in the decision making and play a significant role in the income and expenditure of the family. It appears that, in many sections of the Asian communities, there is a strong desire to continue the extended/joint family system in Britain. One Asian person explained that:

> I have four brothers, all married. Three of us live in one house in this country and one lives with our parents in Pakistan. Our

business, both in Britain and Pakistan, is joint and all the important family and business decisions are taken jointly. We support each other, our children are growing up together in Britain, not just as cousins, but also as friends. We feel more secure and it helps to counter hostility in the wider society against Asians. We would like our children to respect us and look after us when we are old, as we are looking after our parents.

(Interview 1993)

This comment shows that respect for their parents is an important indication for Asians to continue their traditional family system. We compare the information from the 1975 and 1983 surveys in this regard. Both surveys showed (see Table 7.4) that overwhelmingly Asian parents and young people felt that Asian children have more respect for their parents than white children do.

Table 7.4 'Asian children have more respect for their parents than white children do'

Response	Young people		Parents	
	1975 %	1983 %	1975 %	1983 %
Agree	89	80	90	86
Neither agree nor disagree	5	13	6	8
Disagree	6	4	4	*
Don't know	—	3	—	6
Size of sample	1,117	570	1,117	570

Marginally more young people and parents agreed with the statement in 1975 than in 1983, and the number of those who neither agreed nor disagreed increased. However, the number of both young Asians and Asian parents who disagreed with the proposition had actually decreased. Even in this context, many respondents said that it was in the Asian cultures and traditions to respect one's parents and that young Asians were brought up differently from whites, to respect their parents. Three illustrative comments are presented:

Because of our religion. It says, our parents are next to God (in terms of respect) and we respect them.

(Muslim young person 1975)

Some related it to the parents' discipline and what parents do for children to bring them up. A Hindu young person said:

> Because we have been disciplined from the very beginning. The parents do a great deal for you and so you must respect them.

One Asian parent explained:

> Because of our culture, and our children live with parents longer, they see how we have respected our parents and so they learn to respect us as well. White culture is different. Parents themselves may not respect their elders so how can children follow?
>
> (Asian parent 1983)

The last comment is very important and I have heard many Asian parents stressing the fact that some of their traditional way of life could only be transmitted to their children by example. This clearly applies to family relationships. In this context, the prestige of the family is also regarded as being sacrosanct. For example, over 90 per cent of young people took the view that the family and its prestige were important and they would not like to damage the prestige of their families. Some linked it with honour, others felt it was because of their religion. All Asian religious groups were unanimous about the prestige of the family as an important indication of their respect for their parents' religion and traditions.

MARRIAGE

One important aspect of Asian families is the nature of marriage, which binds families together and helps to maintain traditional customs. When a marriage is arranged, it is seen as a contract between the two families and not two individuals, as it is in the Western world. Therefore, the parents and relatives, who arrange a marriage, make sure that it remains intact and use the pressure of family and other relatives, and also sometimes friends, to mediate in case any differences of opinion arise between the husband and wife. However, the result of this depends on whether you marry someone from your own group, where such pressures would work, or you marry somebody from outside the group. In our 1975 and 1983 surveys, we asked both young Asians and parents their attitudes to this question. Their reaction to the statement 'It is better to marry someone from your own group' was very favourable. More

parents (90 per cent) than young people in 1975 favoured endogamy. In 1983, fewer people from both groups agreed with the
statement, but the differences between Asian parents and young
people remained (details are presented in Table 7.5). Parents had
more favourable attitudes to the endogamous marriage than did
young Asians, who, because of their education and experience in
Britain, have a wider outlook and would like to choose marriage
partners on the basis of other individual characteristics.

Table 7.5 'It is better to marry someone from your own group'

	Parents		Young people	
	1975 %	1983 %	1975 %	1983 %
Agree	90	85	78	69
Neither agree nor disagree	3	10	7	20
Disagree	7	1	15	9
Dont know	—	2	—	2
Size of sample	944	212	1,117	570

It is interesting to note that, between 1975 and 1983, the dis-
agreement with the statement amongst Asian parents and young
people had fallen. However, those in the category of 'neither agree
nor disagree' had increased when we compare the results from the
two surveys. Amongst the three religious groups, Muslim and Sikh
young people agreed less with the idea of getting married in one's
own group than their parents did. However, Hindu young people
were least in agreement with the idea compared with their parents.
Those who agreed with the practice of endogamy argued that it was
important to have mutual understanding and knowledge of each
other's way of life. Some believed that marriage is based on religion
and that a mother of the same religion as the father would teach
children about the religion and culture. It appears that more
favourable attitudes amongst Muslims towards endogamy were
also due to the preferential 'cousins' marriage' (preferring to
marry a cousin rather than a non-relative) which is allowed in the
religion. On the other hand, amongst Sikhs and Hindus, marriage
is preferred within the caste or occupational group. Muslims also
consider *Biraderi* (patrilineage, brotherhood, fraternity) relevant in
this context. The argument about customs and religion was
explained by an Asian girl:

> If the husband and wife belong to different groups, it would cause problems with customs and religion; if they belong to your own, no problems afterwards.

Some young Asian people conform to endogamy because of community pressures to the effect that they would otherwise be treated differently and their relationships with their families and relatives could be strained. An Asian young person made a typical comment regarding such pressures:

> If we have a mixed marriage, then we could be outcast from our own people. Relatives will not treat us properly on our side and their side.

Some Asian parents supported the idea of endogamy from their personal experience of happiness and knowledge of the system working very well. However, those who disagreed with the proposition in Table 7.5 mentioned specific reasons, such as personal love and freedom to choose, rather than the importance of the group.

The PSI Survey 1994 (Modood *et al.* 1997) also showed that 'if a close relative were to marry a white person' 51 per cent of Pakistanis, 40 per cent of Bangladeshis, 39 per cent of Indians, and 25 per cent of African Asians said that they would mind a little or very much, compared with only 12 per cent of Caribbean respondents expressing this view. It is worth mentioning that 52 per cent of white respondents would also object to a close relative marrying an ethnic minority person.

Now we turn to the institution of arranged marriages, which receives so much publicity in the British media, often presented as a source of conflict between Asian young people and their parents. However, the empirical evidence suggests that there were still favourable attitudes to arranged marriages, particularly amongst Asian parents. In our survey of 1983, 81 per cent of parents and 58 per cent of young Asians agreed that 'Arranged marriages still work very well within the Asian community and should be continued.' However, agreement on this issue was lower than it was in 1975, when 88 per cent of parents and 67 per cent of young people agreed with the statement. Table 7.6 has full details.

It is interesting to note that, compared with 1975, although fewer young people disagreed in 1983, the percentage of those in the category of 'neither agree nor disagree' has gone up substantially. This could partly be explained by the ambivalent attitudes of young

Table 7.6 'Arranged marriages still work very well within the
Asian community and should be continued'

	Asian parents		Young people	
	1975 %	1983 %	1975 %	1983 %
Agree	88	81	67	58
Neither agree nor disagree	4	9	9	24
Disagree	8	8	24	17
Don't know	—	2	—	2
Size of sample	994	212	1,175	570

people who, although they disagreed with the system of arranged
marriages, were not sure. Therefore, we look at some of the reasons
given by those who agreed and those who disagreed with the
proposition in Table 7.6. The reasons given for supporting
arranged marriages were personal experience and a knowledge
from one's own family that the system had worked well. Many
believed that parents knew what sort of partners their children
would prefer and would find them. One young Asian said, 'because
my parents know my choice, they will pick a good match for me'.
Some argued that the success of arranged marriages could be
judged by looking at the facts, such as that there is usually less
divorce amongst Asians. An Asian parent explained: 'Love marriages are 90 per cent unsuccessful while arranged marriages are
quite OK.' Another Asian parent linked it to age and experience:
'Teenage children cannot judge their future.'

Those who disagreed with the arranged marriage system argued
that young people should be free to choose their own partners. One
Asian father said, 'Times have changed and the Asian community
must march with the times.'

It appears that the custom of arranged marriage is changing,
both in Britain and in the countries of origin. For example, there is
a lot more flexibility and there are various types of discussion
which take place between parents and their children before a decision is taken. Nowadays, it is common for Asians to show photos
of the potential partners to young people, and the young people
can refuse. In some cases, meetings are also arranged between
potential partners by the parents, sometimes in their presence.
There is also a growing number of Asian marriage agencies which
play the role of bringing families together. It is interesting to read

the advertisements of such agencies. Such agencies include the Asha Marriage Bureau, the Suman Marriage Bureau, the International Marriage Bureau, Asian Marriage Lines, and the Muslim Matrimonial. A brief description of these agencies will help to indicate what services they provide.

Asha Marriage Bureau: Do you want to get married to the man or woman of your dreams? Asha ... provides a top class confidential service for parents and independent persons to help you find a suitable marriage partner.

Suman Marriage Bureau: Marriage introductions arranged confidentially by world's largest Asian marriage bureau, established since 1972.

International Marriage Bureau: Most popular world famous match makers. Established since 1984 provides national and international introduction service in a professional manner.

Asian Marriage Lines: Confidential and genuine...phone from anywhere in UK. Hear matrimonial messages of eligible Muslim partners.

The Muslim Matrimonial: Islamic, confidential service (no registration/marriage fee) order latest issues Muslim matrimonial and contact 100s of eligible members...unique new service for British/European Muslims.

These examples are just to indicate that such agencies are now an active part of the Asian communities in areas of high concentration and that they are mainly commercial ventures. In addition, some welfare organisations have also come in to help Asian parents and young people with confidential marriage advice centres. In India, Pakistan and Bangladesh, similar functions are performed by extended family members, friends or traditional '*kami*' caste people, mainly the barbers in rural areas. In urban areas, in addition, some agencies on the lines of the ones mentioned above have also appeared to help families to find suitable partners.

In Britain, several Asian parents now use the Asian press to find suitable partners for their children. There are regular matrimonial columns in Asian magazines and newspapers. These give personal details and indicate what sort of partner is being sought. A few examples will help to illustrate this:

Daughter, 29 years old, successful pharmacist, requires a suitable partner. She is pretty and cultured. Her first marriage ended in divorce. Please respond to this only if you are appropriately educated and have a progressive outlook towards religion and traditions. A telephone no. must be included in the correspondence. (Box No. . . .)

Male, early 30s, 5′ 6″ tall, postgraduate, good looking Sunni Muslim, working as a local government officer in London, earns £19,000 pa, owns a freehold house – looking for a suitable Muslim girl from any nationalities with a view to marriage. (Box No. . . .).

Daughter, British born, smart, beautiful, sophisticated and well versed, aged 24. We are a respectable Asian family. Parents seek a handsome Sunni Muslim gentleman, must be professional or have own business. Photo appreciated. (Box No. . . .)

Male Sunni Muslim from Punjab, Pakistan, 46 years old, British national, smart, own established fashion business, good education very caring – own house, car etc. Seeking a sincere young lady with similar background. Age 38 to 45. Must be active, smart, divorced, widower [*sic*] considered for marriage. (Box No. . . .)

(*Daily Jang*, London, 10 April 1993)

It is clear from the above advertisements that education, religion, national/regional origin and financial security are considered important, in addition to physical characteristics, by Asian parents. My in-depth interviews with Asian parents show that the use of the Asian press and sometimes agencies is a desperate attempt because there is a lack of suitable marriage partners in Britain. It is stressed that, while some Asian boys still prefer to get married in India, Pakistan and Bangladesh, Asian girls are normally reluctant to do that, and this leaves a gap where it is more difficult to find suitable partners for Asian girls. We will return to this problem later in the chapter.

It appears from my research that a growing number of Asian parents, as well as young people, were against the idea of young people's marriages in India, Pakistan or Bangladesh. The main argument used against this idea is that marriages should take place in the community in which young people are brought up. There was also a danger from differences in the educational and cultural background and upbringing of those who live in the Indian subcontinent. So Asians in Britain now feel that the future of young Asians is in Britain and they must try to marry within the Asian community in this country. They feel that there is plenty of choice in Britain and that young people should be able to participate in the decision about their marriage. As indicated above, some Asian parents feel that there is a problem in finding suitable boys for their daughters and therefore they felt forced to look towards the Indian subcontinent. However, my evidence shows that over two-thirds of both Asian parents and young people were against the idea of Asian girls being sent back to the subcontinent to get married. The strong view expressed was that, while Asian girls know the way of life in Britain, they do not know enough about the way of life in the subcontinent. Generally, it appears from Asians girls' attitudes that, as they grow up in Britain, they are more likely to resist being sent back to the subcontinent to get married, even if they have the choice of bringing their husbands to this country.

One way to check on the trend of Asian boys' and girls' marriages being arranged in the Indian subcontinent is to examine the number of male and female fiancé(e)s entering Britain. This method does not give us many details, because some applications by prospective marriage partners are rejected by immigration officers, but it gives some indication of the recent trend. For example, in 1993, 250 male fiancés and 300 female fiancées from the Indian subcontinent were admitted for a limited period for settlement. However, in 1995 this number was reduced to 140 male fiancés and 250 female fiancées from the Indian subcontinent admitted to Britain. This is a downward trend, particularly for Asian girls' marriages being arranged in the subcontinent. Also, due to changes in immigration legislation, fiancé(e)s and newly married couples must serve a probationary period to show marriage was the primary purpose of migration to Britain.

We wanted to know whether parents wanted to keep the system much more than their children did. For this reason, in the 1975 and 1983 surveys, we asked Asian young people and parents about this. In 1975, 85 per cent of the sample, parents and young people alike, agreed that parents wanted to keep arranged marriages more than their children did and only 11 per cent disagreed. Opinions did not vary significantly between religious groups. In 1983, again Asian parents and young people recognised that it was the parents who

wanted to keep the system of arranged marriages (82 per cent
parents and 74 per cent young people). Young people felt that
parents were old-fashioned and more traditional and so wanted
to keep the system of arranged marriages. Parents also believed
that arranged marriages last longer. There were no differences
between young men and women, nor between fathers and mothers,
with respect to their attitudes to arranged marriages. Overall, more
Muslims favoured the idea of arranged marriages than did Hindus
and Sikhs. It is also interesting to point out that middle-class Asian
young people were more likely to accept arranged marriages than
working-class youngsters. There are two explanations for this difference. First, there is more communication between parents and
children in the middle-class families and issues such as marriage are
discussed openly. Second, middle-class parents are more liberal and
have a more flexible and careful approach to the selection of
partners for their children.

It is clear that now Asian children are exposed to the British way
of life, the system of arranged marriages is no longer working in its
rigid form. This view was tested with a proposition in our research
that, 'More and more young people will rebel against arranged
marriages.' The majority of young people (57 and 67 per cent)
agreed with the proposition in both surveys, compared to only a
quarter of parents (24 per cent, in 1983). It is interesting to note
that, in both groups, there was more acceptance of the system in
1983, as fewer believed that young Asians would rebel against
arranged marriages than thought that was the case in 1975. Details
are presented in Table 7.7.

Amongst parents, a majority (57 per cent) thought young people
would rebel in 1975, but, in 1983, only 24 per cent thought they
would. Of all the religious groups, Muslim parents showed the

Table 7.7 'More and more young people will rebel against
arranged marriages'

	Asian young people		Asian parents	
	1975 %	1983 %	1975 %	1983 %
Agree	67	57	57	24
Neither agree nor disagree	11	25	12	33
Disagree	22	16	31	40

highest agreement with the statement (30 per cent), compared to 21 per cent of Hindus and 16 per cent of Sikhs. However, there were no differences between the young people from different religious groups. The two main reasons given by young people for thinking that increasingly young people would rebel against arranged marriages were: (1) people should have the freedom to choose whom they like, and (2) the fact that they now live in a Western society means they should adapt to their new environment. One young Asian commented: 'Asians brought up in this country will behave accordingly and not go back to old traditions.'

Let us now examine how the system of arranged marriages has changed in the last few years.

It is clear from recent evidence that Asian family members play an important role in the selection of a partner. Stopes-Roe and Cochrane (1990) also asked such questions in their study and confirmed this pattern. However, the more recent information about parental involvement in the choice of marriage partner is available from the Fourth National Survey of Ethnic Minorities (Modood *et al.* 1997). It shows, as presented in Table 7.8, that a majority of Indian, Pakistanis and Bangladeshis of age 35 or over had their spouses chosen by their parents. The question posed was: 'What part did your parents play in choosing your husband/wife?'

Table 7.8 Parental involvement in choice of marriage partner (percentages)

Part played	Indian		African Asian		Pakistani		Bangladeshi	
	16–34	35+	16–34	35+	16–34	35+	16–34	35+
Parents made the decision	18	55	9	23	57	68	45	57
I had a say, but parents' decision	9	4	6	8	8	7	5	7
Parents had a say, but my decision	24	11	21	22	15	9	25	12
I talked to my parents, but my decision	27	11	33	22	11	4	6	3
I made decision on my own	20	12	27	22	8	8	8	13
Can't say	3	7	5	3	2	4	11	7

Source: SCPR/PSI Survey 1994 (Modood *et al.* 1997)

It is clear from Table 7.8 that parents' involvement was greatest among Pakistanis and Bangladeshis, and this applied to the 16–34 age group as well. However, the trend for parents' involvement in the Indian and African Asian, 16–34 age groups is declining significantly, with almost one out of four African Asian and one in five Indian young people making their own decisions about their marriage. By comparison, parents made the decisions for 57 per cent of Pakistani and 45 per cent of Bangladeshi young people aged 16–34.

In our 1975 survey, we found that more Muslims (68 per cent) favoured the idea of arranged marriages than did Hindus (51 per cent) and Sikhs (53 per cent). Twenty years later, the 1994 PSI Survey (Modood *et al.* 1997) also found the same trend, as presented in Table 7.9. The statement proposed was: 'The choice of my husband/wife was my parents' decision.' It is clear from this table that the traditional, strict system of arranged marriages is declining for young Asians, However, there are still gender differences, with relatively more Asian young women still conforming to the system.

Table 7.9 Parents' decision over marriage partner, by religious group and age (percentages)

	Hindu		Sikh		Muslim	
Age group	Men	Women	Men	Women	Men	Women
50 + years old	50	74	72	86	62	87
35–49 years old	21	51	49	77	59	78
16–34 years old	18	20	41	27	49	67

Source: SCPR/PSI Survey 1994 (Modood *et al.* 1997)

In the 1970s, arranged marriages were seen as one of the main sources of intergenerational conflict within the Asian communities, but now, with a flexible approach to marriages by parents and with Asian families more settled and confident, fewer see this as an area of rebellion. There is also more consultation and negotiation taking place within Asian families (Modood *et al.* 1997; Stopes-Roe and Cochrane 1990; Anwar 1996). This does not mean that arranged marriages do not create generational conflict in some families, but it is diminishing, particularly now an increasing number of families prefer to arrange their children's marriages in Britain, rather than in Pakistan, Bangladesh or India. Therefore, it appears that the arranged marriages system, with a flexible approach, is likely to continue within Asian communities in Britain in the foreseeable future.

It is worth mentioning here that the ceremonies which take place as part of an Asian wedding in the Indian subcontinent are being organised in a similar way in Britain. Some weddings last up to five days or more, starting with the *Gala*, the official opening of marriage ceremonies, and ending with the *Muklawa*, the consummation of the marriage. They include the *Barat*, the wedding party arrival at the bride's house or place of ceremonies, a community centre or hall, and the *Nikh*, the religious marriage registration. Other ceremonies which take place on the bridegroom's side include *Mehdi*, *Khara Lhoi, Selami* and *Vag Pharai*. There are no doubt variations about the nature and extent of some of these ceremonies, according to the religious affiliation and region of origin of Asians in Britain. However, the point I want to make here is that many Asian families are now confident enough to perform marriage ceremonies in Britain and modify them according to their circumstances. Some ceremonies are performed in a symbolic way (Werbner 1990; Anwar 1979). For example, *Vag Pharai*, the ceremony in which the groom's sister and cousins hold onto the bridle of his horse until he presents them with money, is normally performed in a symbolic way. Another interesting development is that many relatives from the country of origin are also invited to attend weddings in Britain. In some cases, where close relatives of the families involved in the marriage are unable to join, some modified form of smaller ceremonies also takes place in the subcontinent. The reason for this is to show that they too are part of the ceremonies taking place in Britain, thus bringing the British and the country-of-origin ends into a broader context. Those relatives who are unable to participate in the wedding ceremonies in Britain are then sent wedding photographs and a copy of the video, which has become almost an integral part of Asian weddings in Britain. The same applies to weddings of relatives which take place in the subcontinent, where photos and videos of weddings and other important occasions are sent as soon as possible to relatives in Britain who are unable to join such ceremonies. Therefore, it is important to consider the British and subcontinental context as one for marriages and other ceremonies to understand the whole story.

Chapter 8

Religious aspects and the mother tongue

RELIGIOUS ASPECTS

Exposure to Western media and values is one factor which is influencing religious beliefs and attitudes within the Asian communities. Religion is a problematic area, particularly with regard to dress, dietary restrictions, physical and religious education, assembly at school, co-education, etc. Problems in this area are acute amongst Muslims and especially amongst Muslim girls and women, because among Muslims interaction between men and women is limited outside the immediate kin. Also, the sexes are segregated before, or at the time of, puberty. In this section, we examine religious activity and some of the important issues like religious education and single-sex schools, and compare the attitudes and practices of Asian parents and young people.

For many Asians, religion is the main basis for ethnic identity, and it also helps to establish social networks and communicative patterns. Many Asian parents and religious leaders are concerned that not enough facilities are available for them to practise their religion and transmit it to the second and third generations of Asians. There is no doubt that factors such as parental involvement and attitudes and educational influences are very important in the formation of religious knowledge, attitudes and practice. Therefore, sociologists have attached great importance to the notion of socialisation. This means that the transmission of religious culture takes place through the process whereby a child acquires the rules learned through family and friends as well as through organised instruction, i.e. education. However, if family and community members emphasise values that are different from those a child is learning at school, then the child may experience special problems in adapting to life, both in school and at home, and in the community. This is the problem which many Asian children in Britain face. In this context, education cannot be isolated from its social settings, since it is one of the important influences that determines what a child learns. Because of this, Asians generally attach great importance to religious education in schools. The Education Reform Act of 1988 has brought fundamental changes in the education system, including emphasis on Christian assembly and religious education. Many Asian parents are worried about this development.

What it means is that, unless Muslim, Sikh and Hindu parents write to the head teacher of the relevant school stating, 'I do not wish my child to attend Christian collective worship and Christian religious education', the child must attend Christian worship and Christian religious education. It is not clear what happens at schools where a vast majority of children are Muslim, Sikhs or Hindus, regarding Christian worship and Christian religious education. On Christian worship, such schools may get exemption from this provision if the local Standing Advisory Council on Religious Education (SACRE) decides that it would be inappropriate where there is a sizeable number of pupils of non-Christian faiths. However, it appears so far that it is quite difficult to get such an exemption. For these and other reasons, do Asian parents worry about sending their children to predominantly white schools?

In our 1983 survey, four out of six parents and young people disagreed with the proposition that 'Asian parents get very worried about sending their children to predominantly white schools.' However, young Asians were more likely to believe that their parents do get worried (31 per cent) than parents were prepared to admit to being (16 per cent). See Table 8.1 for full details. What were the reasons for their worry?

Table 8.1 'Asian parents get very worried about sending their children to predominantly white schools'

Response	Young Asians %	Asian parents %
Agree	31	16
Neither agree nor disagree	24	43
Disagree	43	40
Size of sample	570	212

Concern about Asians and whites fighting and being able to mix was the main reason for thinking that parents were worried abut their children in white schools. There was also the fear that the children might pick up Western values and ideas. Those who dis-agreed with the proposition did so because they felt the number of white pupils did not make any difference.

One place where Asian religions and cultures could be taught is in schools. In our 1975 survey, 80 per cent of both Asian parents and young people agreed that, 'There is not sufficient formal teaching of Asian religions in English schools', and almost half of the parents (49 per cent) and 41 per cent of young people felt that, 'Children are influenced by Christianity because they attend assemblies at school with a Christian service.' In the 1983 survey, a question was asked about traditional Asian cultures. The majority of all Asian parents and young people believed that there was not enough taught about Asian cultures in schools. See Table 8.2 for full details. One reason for this was thought to be that there were not enough Asian teachers, and, in the main, people felt that things were taught the traditionally British way in traditionally British schools.

Table 8.2 'There is not enough taught about traditional Asian culture in schools'

	Young Asians %	Asian parents %
Agree	66	62
Neither agree nor disagree	20	22
Disagree	9	6
Size of sample	570	212

One Asian parent gave his reason:

My boy does not know how to write his own language. I wish they would teach our language in the school and by way of reading they can learn about our culture as well.

My own recent research has shown that young Asians are also becoming very conscious of the lack of opportunities to learn about their culture within the education system. One young Asian expressed his concern as follows:

We have some facilities to learn about our religion and culture at home and in the community. But I think we should learn about our religion and culture more systematically which we can do at schools. I also want Asian languages to be taught in the schools in the same way and treating them important like German and French. This will also help to read our own books and other religious literature – our cultures should not be treated as a second class compared with English and other European cultures. We are also British and European.

(Asian young person, interview 1994)

This typical comment by a young Asian shows what many Asian young people feel: that their languages and cultures should be treated equally and not as marginal. Asian parents were marginally more concerned about the facilities for practising their religion than young people were. Amongst the religious groups, it appears that Hindus faced more problems than Muslims and Sikhs, who appear to have more mosques and gurdwaras.

In this context, we looked at the religious activity of young Asians and Asian parents. We discovered that, while six out of ten white young people never went to a place of worship, only 28 per cent of Asian young people did not. Similarly, 56 per cent of white young people never prayed, compared with only 18 per cent Asians. Details are presented in Table 8.3.

It is clear from Table 8.3 that a majority (59 per cent) of young Asians pray at least once a week or more often, compared with

Table 8.3 Religious activity of young Asians and young whites

Religious activity	Young Asians %	Young whites %
Praying		
Never	18	56
Once or twice a month or less	20	17
At least once a week	18	6
One or more times a day	41	12
Going to places of worship		
Never	28	60
Once or twice a month or less often	41	24
At least once a week	22	10
One or more times a day	6	*
Size of sample	570	427

Source: 1983 survey

only 18 per cent of white young people. There were also religious differences; for example, half of the young Muslims claimed that they prayed at least once a day. Ghuman (1994) also found young Muslims more conservative than Sikhs and Hindus. When we compare Asian parents with young people, however, we see that the parents prayed more often, as shown in Table 8.4.

Table 8.4 Religious activity of Asian parents any young Asians

	Young Asians %	Asian parents %
Praying		
Never	18	2
Once or twice a month or less often	20	7
At least once a week	18	10
One or more times a day	41	77
Going to places of worship		
Never	28	19
Once or twice a month or less often	41	30
At least once a week	22	33
One or more times a day	6	15
Size of sample	570	212

Source: 1983 survey

Similarly, Asian parents were also more likely to attend a place of worship than younger people were. Once again, Muslim parents were more likely to say their prayers one or more times a day than were Hindus and Sikhs, partly because Muslims are obliged to pray five times a day. It is clear from my more recent research that a lot of young Asians go to religious services not only to please their families, but also because they like praying and participating in religious observance. However, they also feel that their parents had the advantage of more religious teaching than they have had. Many young people complained that facilities for prayers were not available at school.

The importance of religion and attendance of religious service was also covered in the Fourth PSI Survey (Modood *et al.* 1997). Once again, the earlier trend was confirmed and the survey showed that Muslims were more likely (74 per cent) than Hindus (43 per cent) and Sikhs (46 per cent) to say that religion was very important in the way they lived their life. Table 8.5 shows the details of

Table 8.5 Importance of religion (percentages)

Response	Hindu	Sikh	Muslim	Church of England		Roman Catholic		Old Protestant		New Protestant
				White	Other	White	Other	White	Other	Caribbeans*
Very important	43	46	74	11	37	32	35	32	43	71
Fairly important	46	40	21	35	32	37	38	30	42	24
Not important	11	14	4	53	30	32	27	38	15	5
Weighted count	453	410	677	1,379	164	317	89	198	129	138
Unweighted count	419	363	1,033	1,395	131	317	75	201	102	101

Source: SCPR/PSI Survey 1994 (Modood et al. 1997)
* The non-Caribbean New Protestants were too few for analysis.
Base: Those who have a religion

Table 8.6 Attendance at religious service (percentages)

Response	Hindu	Sikh	Muslim	Church of England		Roman Catholic		Old Protestant		New Protestant Caribbeans*
				White	Other	White	Other	White	Other	
Once a week or more	27	39	62	9	30	29	26	28	25	57
Once a month but less than once a week	24	32	7	7	13	12	16	11	28	17
Once a year but less than once a month	29	19	6	38	36	29	30	31	31	15
Less than once a year	18	7	17	45	30	29	21	30	13	9
Can't say	3	2	7	—	—	1	6	1	3	1
Weighted count	453	410	677	1,379	164	317	89	198	129	138
Unweighted count	419	363	1,033	1,395	131	317	75	201	102	101

Source: SCPR/PSI Survey 1994 (Modood et al. 1997)
* The non-Caribbean New Protestants were too few for analysis.

the sample, which also covers other religious groups. The question posed was: 'How important is religion to the way you live your life?'

One other group which shows a pattern similar to Muslims in the table is that of New Protestant Caribbeans, who saw religion as very important in their lives. It is worth pointing out that very few white people in the Church of England (11 per cent) saw religion as very important.

Let us now see how these attitudes translate into behaviour. Once again, the overall pattern of religious groups does not change significantly, as presented in Table 8.6. The question posed was: 'How often do you attend services or prayer meetings or go to a place of worship?'

The survey also showed that, for all religious groups, the younger generation were less likely to attend, which confirms the trend discovered in our 1975 and 1983 surveys.

One other issue which has a religious angle is single-sex schools. The issue of separate schools for Muslims has recently received a lot of press coverage. Some commentators have confused this with the genuine demands of Muslims and other parents who would like to send their children to single-sex schools. The 1983 survey showed that a majority of Muslims, both parents and young people, and Sikh parents agreed that Asian parents would like to send their daughters to single-sex schools, whereas a minority of Hindus, both parents and young people, and young Sikhs favoured them (see Table 8.7 for details). Whilst there has been no change in the attitudes of Muslim parents on this issue since the 1975 survey

Table 8.7 'Asian parents would like to send their daughters to single-sex schools'

Response	Young Asians				Asian parents			
	All %	Muslim %	Hindu %	Sikh %	All %	Muslim %	Hindu %	Sikh %
Agree	50	68	39	40	63	76	39	62
Neither agree nor disagree	26	17	30	33	17	16	28	9
Disagree	4	12	29	23	15	8	19	26
Per cent agreeing in 1975	60	80	45	52	65	83	50	57
Size of sample	570	219	200	123	212	92	54	58

(83 per cent agreed), young Muslims were less likely to agree with the proposition in 1983 (68 per cent) than in 1975 (80 per cent).

The differences in attitudes between Muslims and Hindus and Sikhs are quite clear from Table 8.7. The main reason for thinking that Asian parents would prefer to send girls to single-sex schools was that it would be morally wrong to do otherwise. Most of those who held this view also agreed that they did not like girls mixing with boys. One parent explained:

> Co-education is OK until they are teenagers then the problems start about going out with boys etc. because we like our girls to marry in our own religious groups and see them happy.

Another father said:

> It is the religion, girls should not mix with boys.

Many parents expressed anxiety at the permissiveness, as they saw it, of British society in general and young people in particular.

The issue of single-sex schools is not a new one. The Swann Committee (1985) also recommended that where there is parental concern about the education of girls, existing co-educational schools with multi-racial pupil populations could do more to ensure that, in certain specific areas, separate provision is offered on a single-sex basis, as appropriate, in the school's activities. It added 'we hope that LEAs with a multi-racial pupil population will consider carefully the value of retaining an option of single-sex education as part of their school provision' (Swann 1985). A Muslim Charter of Demands issued by several national and regional Muslim organisations in 1987 also included continuance of single-sex schools for boys and girls as part of the state school system. In fact, the development of some independent Muslim schools is partly due to Muslim parents' worries about the non-availability of single-sex schools for their girls, as such schools are fast disappearing. There are currently fifty-three Muslim independent schools in England and Wales and none is yet receiving government funding.

The Fourth PSI survey (Modood et al. 1997) also included a few questions about preferences for single-sex schools and religious schools. It showed that the majority of Pakistani respondents preferred single-sex schools for their daughters, and the pattern of responses was similar for 16–34-year-old young people (see Table 8.8 for details). There was also significant minority support among

Table 8.8 Preference for single-sex schooling for one's daughters and sons (percentages)

Schooling preference	White		Irish		Caribbean		Indian		African Asian		Pakistani		Bangladeshi		Chinese	
	Daughters	Sons	Daughters	Sons	Daughters	Sons	Daughters	Sons	Daughters	Sons	Daughters	Sons	Daughters	Sons	Daughters	Sons
Single-sex	19	16	29	27	19	12	26	17	23	19	59	27	46	33	29	17
Mixed	52	55	44	51	52	58	36	41	33	34	16	33	12	18	32	35
No preference	26	26	26	22	26	27	34	38	40	42	20	35	29	36	34	42
Can't say	3	3	0	0	4	3	5	4	5	5	6	5	13	13	5	5
Weighted count	2,757		110		147		784		442		408		646		196	
Unweighted count	2,748		119		302		591		601		378		635		110	
Preference for single-sex amongst 16–34-year-olds	10	7	22	18	19	10	19	12	17	15	48	19	37	27	21	10

Source: SCPR/PSI Survey 1994 (Modood et al. 1997)

other Asian groups, particularly in a preference for single-sex schooling for their daughters. The Irish and Chinese showed a significant preference for such schooling too. The white and Caribbean respondents were least likely to show preferences for their sons or daughters to go to single-sex schools.

Let us now examine the respondents' attitudes to schools of one's own religion. Although Muslims receive more publicity for having a preference for schools based on their own religion, in fact more support came from Roman Catholics for such schools, as shown in Table 8.9.

The pattern of support for such schools for all religious groups among young people was not any different, except that only 1 per cent of Sikhs supported them. However, more Sikhs without qualifications supported such schools (21 per cent) than among Hindus (11 per cent). A similar pattern applied to Muslims, although a relatively larger proportion with A-levels or higher qualifications (18 per cent) gave a preference for schools of one's own religion than among Hindus (3 per cent) and Sikhs (2 per cent).

The question arises of how these schools based on one's own religion should be funded. There are currently over 4,500 denominational schools funded by the government as voluntary-aided schools. However, after several attempts by Muslim schools to get such a status with government funding, as mentioned above, at the time of writing no Muslim school had succeeded. There appears to be support for religious schools within the state sector among some religious groups as revealed by the Fourth PSI Survey (Modood *et al.* 1997), presented in Table 8.10. The statement proposed was: 'There should be state schools for people belonging to particular religions.'

It is interesting to note that the lowest support for religious schools within the state sector came from the Hindu respondents (12 per cent) and the maximum support was found among the Muslim respondents (48 per cent). In fact this reflects the concerns of Muslims for the lack of such state support, and some Muslims see this as discriminatory because Christian and Jewish schools are already receiving state financial support for denominational schools.

One of the reasons for the development of, and demand for, Muslim independent schools is because some Muslim parents prefer to send their daughters, in particular, to single-sex schools, and this is confirmed by the empirical evidence presented above. The

Table 8.9 Preference for schools of one's own religion (percentages)

Preference for school of one's own religion	Hindu	Sikh	Muslim	Church of England		Roman Catholic		Old Protestant		New Protestant
				White	Other	White	Other	White	Other	Other
All	6	9	28	17	11	38	37	12	13	30
16–34-year-olds	9	1	23	13	10	34	24	15	15	30
Persons without qualifications	11	21	35	20	10	36	37	9	5	26
Persons with A-levels or higher education	3	2	18	14	13	41	45	11	23	37

Source: SCPR/PSI Survey 1994 (Modood et al. 1997)

Table 8.10 Support for religious schools within the state sector (percentages)

Response	Persons without religion		Hindu	Sikh	Muslim	Church of England		Roman Catholic		Old Protestant		New Protestant
	White	Other				White	Other	White	Other	White	Other	Other
Yes	23	22	12	20	48	26	21	41	35	20	20	36
No	69	62	72	61	28	64	70	50	57	71	67	51
Can't say	8	17	15	19	24	10	9	9	8	9	13	13

Source: SCPR/PSI Survey 1994 (Modood et al. 1997)

other reason is the lack of religious facilities and of opportunities for children to learn about their religion.

THE MOTHER TONGUE

Some Asian parents have also expressed their concern about the non-availability of mother-tongue teaching, which they see as an integral part of their religion and culture. There is no doubt that mother-tongue skills help to give access to Asian religions and cultures, because a lot of their literature is in those languages.

There seems to be a view in schools that any language used at home other than English hinders the process of learning English at school. This applies to Asians but it is contested by experts in the field. In 1975, when asked whether they spoke their mother tongue at home, 91 per cent of parents and 85 per cent of children claimed that they spoke their mother tongue instead of English. There was a relationship between the age of young people on arrival in Britain and the use of the mother tongue. Gujarati and Bengali speakers were marginally more likely to use their mother tongue than those whose main language was Punjabi, Hindi or Urdu. In most cases, young people claimed that they spoke the mother tongue because there was someone in the household who did not understand English. It is relevant to point out that, in the 1983 survey, the pattern of the use of the mother tongue at home had not changed in any significant way compared to 1975. However, the reasons were different. For example, in 1983, in addition to the communication reason, more young persons gave religio-cultural reasons. They felt that one way to keep their cultures alive in Britain was to keep learning their mother tongue or 'community languages'. A significant number of Asian parents and young people now feel that Asian languages should be treated as part of the school curriculum in the same way as European languages. This feeling was shared by many young people who feel proud of their mother tongue and see it as part of their ethnic and cultural identity.

It is perhaps due to cultural identity or to communication between parents and children that most of the Asian young people spoke their mother tongue at home. To see how the pattern had changed over time we compared the results of the 1975 and 1983 surveys. Respondents were asked whether they could talk and understand English as well as their mother tongue. Eighty-five per cent of young Asian people in 1975 claimed to understand English as well

Table 8.11 'I find that I can talk and understand English as well as my mother tongue', 1975

| Response | All parents % | All young people % | Parents | | ABC1 parents % | ABC1 young people % | C2DE parents % | C2DE young people % |
			Male %	Female %				
Agree	49	85	66	30	65	87	44	85
Neither agree nor disagree	3	2	3	4	4	1	3	2
Disagree	48	13	31	66	31	12	53	13
Size of sample	944	1,117	587	358	256	300	601	702

Source: 1975 survey

as their mother tongue. On the other hand, only 49 per cent of parents made this claim and 48 per cent did not, as shown in Table 8.11. There was no difference between the answers of boys and girls; nor between young people born in Britain or those who arrived at different ages. However, looking at parents, only 31 per cent of men did not speak English compared with 66 per cent of women.

As shown in Table 8.11, middle-class parents as well as young people claimed that they spoke more English than working-class parents. Speaking English did not relate to specific mother tongues except in the case of Bengali speakers, who were less likely to be proficient in English. This is partly due to their rural backgrounds and partly because of more recent arrival in Britain, as pointed out in Chapter 1.

In the 1983 survey, we again found that young Asians were more likely to talk and understand English as well as their mother tongue than parents were. However, there seems to be a small decline among both parents and young people in this respect (see Table 8.12 for details). It appears that marginally more parents spoke and understood English, due to their longer stay in Britain, and fewer young Asians could talk and understand their mother tongue, due to lack of facilities to learn their language and pressures from 'experts' or parents to speak to their children in English at home. For example, 8 per cent of young people born in Britain claimed not to speak English as well as their mother tongue. Half (49 per cent) of the Asian parents who had arrived in this country in the 1960s still did not speak English as well as their mother tongue.

Table 8.12 'I find I can talk and understand English as well as my mother tongue', 1983

Response	Young Asians %	Parents %
Agree	80	31
Neither agree nor disagree	5	11
Disagree	12	52
Size of sample	570	212

Those who arrived in the 1970s showed a similar pattern, except that 58 per cent disagreed with the statement. Altogether, just over half of Asian parents could not understand English well, which means that children spoke their mother tongue at home to communicate with their parents. On the whole, this confirmed the assumption that a significant proportion of first generation Asians still faced language and communication difficulties. This applies in particular to Asian women. These trends were also confirmed by a national survey of racial minorities in 1982. It showed that, while 21 per cent of Asian men spoke English 'slightly' or 'not at all', 47 per cent of Asian women were in this situation. In particular, of those who spoke English 'not at all', 20 per cent were women as against only 4 per cent of Asian men. Two groups of women with a lack of English were worth noting; Bangladeshi women (76 per cent) and Pakistani women (70 per cent), who spoke either little English or none at all (Brown 1984).

It is also worth testing here the point I made above that many Asians are in favour of preserving their mother tongue. The Third PSI Survey (Brown 1984) showed that there was an overwhelming (95 per cent) support for this. Asians were also asked whether 'Children should be taught the language of the family's area of origin.' Ninety-four per cent of all Asians agreed with the statement. As is clear from Table 8.13, relatively more Pakistanis and African Asians 'agreed strongly with the statement'.

There was little difference in attitudes between the young and old respondents or between those who had fluent English and poor English. It is clear that Asian parents and young people would like to preserve their country-of-origin languages, and therefore their criticisms of the education system for not providing facilities to learn their languages as part of school curriculum provision need to be taken seriously by the relevant authorities.

Table 8.13 'Children should be taught the language of the family's area of origin'

	All Asians %	Indians %	Pakistanis %	Bangladeshis %	African Asians %
Agree strongly	55	48	62	51	60
Agree	39	43	34	39	37
Neither agree nor disagree	3	4	2	5	1
Disagree	2	3	1	4	1
Disagree strongly	1	1	—	1	1

Source: Brown 1984

One recent survey (Rudat 1994) showed that Indians were more likely to speak English (32 per cent) as their main language of conversation, compared with Pakistanis (22 per cent) and Bangladeshis (10 per cent). Punjabi was the main language of nearly half of Pakistanis and a quarter of Indians, and 36 per cent of Indians used Gujarati as their main language for conversation. Almost

Table 8.14 Main languages spoken, 1992 (percentages)

Group/language	%
Indian	
Gujarati	36
English	32
Punjabi	24
Urdu	3
Hindi	2
Other	3
All languages	100
Pakistani	
Punjabi	48
Urdu	24
English	22
Other	6
All languages	100
Bangladeshi	
Bengali	73
Sylheti	17
English	10
All languages	100

Source: Rudat 1994

three out of four Bangladeshis said that their main spoken language was Bengali, with a further 17 per cent who said it was Sylheti (which is a dialect of Bengali), as shown in Table 8.14.

The survey showed that the main language spoken varied with age. For example, more 16–29-year-old Indians and Pakistanis in the sample said that they spoke English as their main language. In all three Asian ethnic groups the proportion who spoke English as their main language decreased with age. Only 20 per cent of Indian men and just under 10 per cent of Indian women, and virtually no Bangladeshis aged 50–74, said that English was their main spoken language.

The Fourth PSI Survey (Modood *et al.* 1997) also asked questions about the use of South Asian languages. It showed that an overwhelming majority of Asians spoke a non-European language and a majority of them were also able to write it, as shown in Table 8.15.

Table 8.15 Persons who speak and write a non-European language in Britain (percentages)

	Indian	African Asian	Pakistani	Bangladeshi
Speak	88	92	92	97
Write	58	60	58	85

Source: SCPR/PSI Survey 1994 (Modood *et al.* 1997)

A further analysis showed that among the four ethnic groups the majority of Indians spoke Punjabi, as did Pakistanis, the majority of African Asians spoke Gujarati, and the majority of Bangladeshis spoke Bengali as well as Sylheti. See Table 8.16 for details.

It must be pointed out, however, that some Asians spoke more than one Asian language and, therefore, there is an overlap between different ethnic groups in the use of community languages mentioned in Table 8.16. Interesting findings from the survey relate to age; these showed that, while nearly all the younger generation 16–34-year-olds still sometimes use a community language in talking to family members older than themselves, only about half of Indians and African Asians, six out of ten Pakistanis and a high 85 per cent of Bangladeshis in this age group used an Asian language with family members of their own age group (Modood *et al.* 1997). While the situational use of Asian languages varies with age group, overall, the pattern of language use among young

Table 8.16 Use of Asian languages (percentages)

Language use	Indian	African Asian	Pakistani	Bangladeshi
Hindi				
Speaks	33	44	5	22
With younger family	5	3	—	—
Gujarati				
Speaks	20	67	—	—
With younger family	17	44	—	—
Punjabi				
Speaks	62	30	74	4
With younger family	43	17	51	1
Urdu				
Speaks	13	18	73	21
With younger family	4	3	41	3
Bengali				
Speaks	2	1	—	56
With younger family	1	—	—	42
Sylheti				
Speaks	—	1	—	60
With younger family	—	—	—	55

Source: Adapted from SCPR/PSI Survey 1994 (Modood *et al.* 1997)

Asians did not differ significantly compared to what we found in our survey of 1983, presented in Table 8.12.

There are indications that, while many Asian children are able to speak their mother tongue or community languages, they are not in the same way proficient in reading and writing these languages. However, for access to religious and cultural literature in Asian languages, reading is important. Therefore, in Asian communities, many supplementary schools or classes are arranged to teach Asians not only their religion and religious practice, but also their community or heritage languages. Such provision is generally attached to mosques, gurdwaras and temples. These classes are held either after school hours or at weekends. However, many Asian parents and young people would like such a provision as part of the school curriculum. Young Asians have shown that they wished to learn to read and write their mother tongue and would like to pass it on to their children (Ghuman 1994; Drury 1991). In one study of 16–20-year-olds, 72 per cent of Sikh young people would have liked to study Punjabi at school and 95 per cent of the respondents hoped to pass it on to their children (Drury 1991). These findings are consistent with the ones analysed above from the 1975, 1983 and 1994 surveys. There is also a significant desire among Asians that public libraries should keep books in Asian languages to provide a facility for those who cannot speak English, to keep Asians in touch with their traditional cultures, and to keep people in practice with their community language. In this context, Asian-language newspapers and radio programmes also reinforce this linguistic importance in addition to providing information and entertainment.

It is clear from the discussion and analysis in this chapter that Asians would like to preserve their religions and mother tongues as they see these as an integral part of their ethnic and cultural identity. It is also clear that the second generation Asians would like not only to learn to read and write in relevant Asian languages but also to pass this on to their children. The same applies to their religion and religious practices. There also seems to be a desire that, in addition to the community facilities to teach religion and languages, schools should teach these as part of the school curriculum. Smith and Tomlinson (1989) also found that the majority of all second generation Asians wanted a greater recognition and teaching of their religion in schools.

There is a widespread feeling among Asians that their religions and languages are not treated by the education system in the same way as Christianity and European languages such as French, German, Spanish, etc. It appears that Asian parents' pressures are likely to increase for equal treatment in this context. Every study in the last twenty years of Asian young people has concluded that, despite the indications of generational gap within Asian communities, religion is seen as part of their distinctive ethnic identity (Anwar 1976; Brah 1978; Stopes-Roe and Cochrane 1990; Drury 1991; Ghuman 1994: Modood *et al.* 1994). Religion and related aspects are seen as a fundamental part of their daily lives and as the core of their ethnic identity. This is evident from the generous financial contributions which are made for the construction and running of mosques, gurdwaras and temples, up and down Britain. There are also numerous local, regional and national religious organisations which arrange religious activities for their communities and therefore help the practice and transmission of religion in and to the current and future generations. To conclude, it is clear that religion and Asian languages are likely to play their symbolic and actual role in the foundation of ethnic identities in the Asian communities in the foreseeable future.

It is important to point out that this pattern is not peculiar to Asians in Britain. Jews have used their synagogues as a major institution for identification with Judaism and the Hebrew language. Poles in this country belong to separate Polish Roman Catholic parishes. The Irish in Britain generally follow the Roman Catholic church, and this has played an important part in preserving an Irish ethnic identity.

It appears that some of the religious activities of Asians are seen by white Christian people, and sometimes presented by the media, as alien, due to differences in outlook and behaviour. Such behaviour sometimes appears as the cause of conflict with white people. The Rushdie affair is a good example in this context, but also, several problems have arisen regarding Asian places of worship in several areas. Diversity is seen by some sections of the white community as threatening and 'Asians taking over'. However, the reality is quite different. They are trying to practise their religions and to transmit them to the next generation as an integral part of their ethnic and cultural identities.

Chapter 9

Leisure, freedom and clothes

It is now well known that most Asians, for social and cultural reasons, spend their spare time with other Asians. Some do this because of language difficulties. An additional reason is that, in this way, they avoid hostility and rejection from white people. In our research, we wanted to know whether Asians wanted to be with other Asians in their spare time, and also whether they enjoyed living in areas where there were lots of other Asian families. These indications could also show attitudes towards inter-ethnic relations. In this section, we present the results from the 1975, 1983 and 1994 surveys, which also cover issues of leisure, freedom and the meaning of Asian and Western clothes.

BEING WITH OTHER ASIANS

Respondents were asked whether they wanted to be with other Asians in their spare time. Whilst the majority of Asian parents wanted to be with other Asians for most of their spare time, less than half of young Asians felt the same. The main reason for agreeing with this statement (see Table 9.1) was that they (young people and parents) liked to be with people who had the same background. Parents in the 1983 survey were more likely to want to spend their leisure time with other Asians than in 1975 (up from 65 per cent in 1975 to 74 per cent in 1983). Full details are presented in Table 9.1.

The differences in attitudes of young Asians who disagreed with the statement between the 1975 and 1983 samples are significant. In this, as in many other aspects covered in this book, the main reasons for differences in attitudes seemed to be social class and religion. Parents, particularly Asian mothers, would like to be with

Table 9.1 'I want to be with other Asians for most of my spare time'

Response	Asian parents		Young people	
	1975 %	1983 %	1975 %	1983 %
Agree	65	74	47	43
Neither agree nor disagree	11	16	14	29
Disagree	24	5	39	25

other Asians more than the young people would. Working-class respondents (C2DE), both parents and young people, wanted to spend their spare time with other Asians more than the middle-class respondents (ABC1) did. Also, among religious groups, more Muslim young people preferred to spend their spare time with other Asians than young people of Sikh and Hindu religious groups. The main reason, particularly amongst Asian parents, seemed to be the ease of communication within the Asian group and sometimes a lack of ability to communicate with English-speaking people. There is also less formality involved and people find it more relaxing within their own group. Nevertheless, several Asian respondents thought that Asian people should mix socially with all sections of the community. What is clear is that Asians, like other groups, wanted to spend their spare time with other members of the same group. However, this tended to be less true of Asian young people, who had more opportunities to meet white and other young people than did their parents, whose exposure to the white population was limited. Young Asians also did not have language difficulties. This means that, as more Asian children grow up in Britain, there will be more chance to create friendships across ethnic boundaries, at least in theory. However, both Asian parents and young people still faced hostility and sometimes discrimination from some sections of the white population, which discourages inter-ethnic friendships. In this context, we wanted to test their attitudes to living in an Asian-concentration area.

It appeared that Asian parents were also more likely to enjoy living in an area where there were lots of other Asian families than Asian young people. For example, 70 per cent agreed with this compared to 48 per cent of young people (see Table 9.2).

Those parents and young people who agreed with this view thought that it was easier to make friends with people from the

Table 9.2 'I enjoy living in an area where there are a lot of other Asian families'

Reponse	Asian parents %	Young people %
Agree	70	48
Neither agree nor disagree	22	29
Disagree	5	21
Size of sample	212	570

Source: 1983 survey

same background and that it was nice to have friends and relatives close by. The following qualitative comments help to illustrate some of these points:

> I like to live in my community and I like to live with my own people. I enjoy the attitudes and festivals of our culture.
>
> (Asian parent)

> If you have a lot of Asian people living nearby then you can discuss problems because everybody has the same problems and you can visit them.
>
> (Young Asian)

> I do not feel foreigner living with people of my own background.
>
> (Young Asian)

In my recent research in Birmingham, respondents had put a greater emphasis on community and places of worship including supplementary schools in the areas of Asian concentrations. They valued these facilities and Asian shops, which made a difference to their daily lives, as one respondent explained:

> I think we are more at ease in living in an area like Small Heath, where we have almost every facility a community needs, shops, mosques, Muslim schools, Urdu newspapers, travel agents, etc. Even the local state schools, in practice, have 90 per cent Asian children. There is a real and thriving community and we feel safer here than I would in a predominantly white area. It is good for our children to grow up with these community facilities available.
>
> (Asian parent, interview 1994)

A young Asian explained the benefits of living in an 'Asian area' in this way:

We used to live in Wolverhampton in a council housing flat in an area with a lot of white gangs. As a child I was beaten up several times by white boys and girls. Since we moved to Birmingham in 1982 and started living in this area [Sparkbrook] our outlook towards living in Britain has changed. I remember, at one point, that my father wanted to go back to Pakistan and, after moving here [Birmingham], we are so happy that he has never mentioned this recently. We have everything we need in the area within walking distance. In fact, as a result of competition between relatives, my education and that of my brothers and sisters has improved. We have also benefited from the religious education facilities and I can go on and on about the benefits of the area.

(Young Asian, interview 1994)

It is clear from the above qualitative answers that Asian people generally valued living in Asian-concentration areas. However, some also complain about the bad physical conditions of houses and the quality of schools and leisure facilities in some of these inner-city areas. Some leisure activities no doubt still take place outside these areas, and in this context now we turn to the issues of freedom and leisure activities.

LEISURE AND FREEDOM

It is true that Asian parents' restrictions can cause conflict between parents and children wishing to adapt to Western freedom and leisure activities. Many of these restrictions are normally directed at limiting the opportunities for the sexes to mix. Asian parents generally feel that their children, girls in particular, must be protected from forming any undesirable relationships. It is generally accepted by Asian young people that white children of their own age have more freedom. They also admit that Asian parents disapprove of Western ways, such as having boyfriends or girlfriends. Some young Asians feel frustrated because they would like to have more freedom than their parents would give them. In the 1975 survey, young Asians were asked whether they 'would like more freedom than parents give them'. A minority (35 per cent) of young people agreed with the proposition, while 58 per cent disagreed. Asian girls more often than boys felt they would like more freedom. Working-class young people wanted more freedom than middle-class young Asians did. The same patterns emerged in the follow-up research on this issue. One explanation about the class differences could be that working-class Asian parents are more conservative in their outlook but their children are not. The parents' rural backgrounds and lack of higher education may make them more restrictive than middle-class Asian parents, who are better educated and tend to be more liberal in their views and more flexible in their approach to giving freedom to their children.

Since we were interested in comparing Asian parents' attitudes with those of young people, we found that the reasons given by those who would like more freedom certainly showed a generation gap. However, some of those who did not want more freedom felt that too much freedom given to children at a young age could spoil them.

Looking to the future, it appears that a majority of young people would allow much more freedom to their children than they had. Asian girls, in particular, on the basis of their personal experience of what they considered over-harsh restrictions, would like to give more freedom to their children. There seems to be a growing feeling that young Asian people should have more independence and freedom so that they can learn to stand on their own feet. In sum, it appears that patterns of restriction and freedom are likely to change with the successive generations of Asians in Britain.

As indicated above, more restrictions are placed on the freedom of women and girls than of boys in the Asian communities; therefore, we explored whether our respondents would allow their teenage daughters to go to the same places as white girls. There were substantial differences in the attitudes of parents and young people and between older and younger children. Only a minority of young people in every age and religious group, except Muslims, agreed with the proposition in Table 9.3, while the majority of parents in

Table 9.3 'If I had teenage daughters I would not let them go to any of the places where white girls go to in this area'

	Asian parents		Young people	
Response	1975 %	1983 %	1975 %	1983 %
Agree	57	44	38	31
Neither agree nor disagree	9	25	13	19
Disagree	34	29	49	49

all groups agreed with it. It is also interesting to point out that mothers and fathers shared similar views on this.

It is clear from Table 9.3 that attitudes had become more tolerant since 1975. Thirty-eight per cent of young people and 57 per cent of parents then agreed that they would restrict the activities of their teenage daughters, compared to 31 per cent and 44 per cent respectively in 1983. Two comments in this context are relevant to quote:

> We like children to keep our culture and not get Westernised and for them to be unhappy.
>
> (Asian parent 1983)

> English girls go out with boyfriends and it teaches Asian to do the same.
>
> (Young Asian 1983)

Asian parents, and Muslims in particular, were protective about their daughters: 44 per cent of all Asian parents in the 1983 survey, and 54 per cent of Muslims, agreed that they would not let their teenage daughters go to places where white girls go. However, generally fewer young Asians were in favour of restricting the activities of teenage girls. Only 31 per cent of all young people agreed with the statement. Agreement was higher amongst young Muslims (45 per cent) than other religious groups (Sikhs 26 per cent, Hindus 23 per cent). The fact that 'their religion would not allow it' and the 'lack of morals' amongst white girls were the two main reasons for not allowing their daughters to go to places with white girls. It is interesting to note that young women (54 per cent) and mothers (32 per cent) were more likely to disagree with the statement than young men (44 per cent) and fathers (26 per cent). It is, however, clear that Muslims, both parents and young people, felt most strongly on this subject. This trend was confirmed in my more recent research on Muslims. Their reasons were mainly cultural and religious. For example, it was argued that dancing, which is one of the main leisure activities of white girls, is forbidden in Islam. There was also the extended family and community pressure for Asian girls to be 'modest' in their behaviour and dress. The wearing of Western dress by Asian girls was also seen as indicative of freedom. Therefore, we now examine Asian parents' attitudes towards Asian girls wearing Western clothes and compare these with the attitudes of young Asians.

CLOTHES

Dress often distinguishes Asians from the rest of the society. This applies largely, but not solely, to Muslim women and girls, who traditionally must be covered from head to foot, and this can cause problems in the school and other institutions. For example, in schools, Muslim girls above a certain age are unable to wear shorts for games or use swimming costumes in mixed swimming pools. Some Muslim girls have been refused professional training, such as nursing, or employment because of their traditional dress. Some schools and employers also object to Muslim girls or women wearing *Hijab* (head scarves). There are also conflicts within Asian families when young people refuse to wear Asian clothes, because they want to adopt the Western style of dress and their parents do not want them to. Western dress is also seen as a gesture of more freedom by young people.

The majority of young Asians (65 per cent) did not see anything wrong with Asian girls wearing Western clothes, although less than half of parents (44 per cent) held this view and 27 per cent disagreed with it. Among both young people and parents, females are the most likely to see nothing wrong with Asian girls wearing Western clothes, as presented in Table 9.4.

Table 9.4 'I do not see anything wrong with Asian girls wearing Western clothes'

	Asian young people			Asian parents		
	All %	Men %	Women %	All %	Men %	Women %
Agree	65	59	71	44	41	48
Neither agree nor disagree	16	19	12	27	30	24
Disagree	18	20	16	27	27	28
Size of sample	570	302	268	212	115	97

Source: 1983 survey

Young people did not see anything wrong with wearing Western clothes, mainly because they lived in a Western society and it would help them fit in better. There was also a feeling that girls should be free to wear what they wanted. Others mentioned that clothes were not important and made no difference to cultural traditions. On the other hand, religion was given as the main reason for thinking that girls should not wear Western clothes. It is also worth mentioning that opposition amongst parents to young girls wearing Western clothes was less in 1983 (27 per cent) than in 1975 (38 per cent).

Another question was asked to discover parents' and young Asians' attitudes to whether most Asian girls would like to wear more Western clothes. Almost twice as many young Asians (60 per cent) as parents (35 per cent) agreed with the statement (see Table 9.5 for details). It is interesting to note that significantly fewer Asian parents in 1983 thought that girls wanted to wear Western clothes (35 per cent) than in 1975 (62 per cent). Young Asian women and mothers were more likely to agree with the statement than men. The main reason given for thinking that most Asian girls would like to wear Western clothes was that it would help them to mix in more easily and that they were more fashionable and comfortable.

Table 9.5 'Most Asian girls would like to wear more Western clothes'

	Asian young people			Asian parents		
	All %	Men %	Women %	All %	Men %	Women %
Agree	60	58	61	35	29	41
Neither agree nor disagree	28	30	24	41	46	35
Disagree	12	10	13	23	23	23

Source: 1983 survey

It is worth pointing out that there had also been a slight decrease amongst those young people who thought girls would like to wear Western clothes between 1983 (60 per cent) and 1975 (69 per cent). One Asian girl explained her support this way:

In this country we have to live up to their standards. I do not wish to be different – keeping in fashion.

Asian girls themselves held the view in favour of Western clothes more strongly than boys. On the whole Muslims emerged as the most conservative group. This has been found in other studies as well (Evans 1971; Ballard 1994; Modood *et al.* 1994). Partly it is because of religion and partly because, comparatively, the majority of Muslims are more recent arrivals than are Hindus and Sikhs. In addition, as shown in Chapter 2, more Muslims are working-class with rural backgrounds than is true of other Asian religious groups. Several respondents also commented that Western clothes were not decent and skirts and other 'funny naked dresses' exposed the body too much, of which Asian communities do not approve. Finally, it is clear that opinions on this matter were divided within and between generations and on gender lines, and have a potential for conflict within Asian families.

The Fourth PSI Survey (Modood *et al.* 1997) also asked questions about the wearing of Asian clothes, and the findings confirmed the pattern of attitudes to the wearing of Asian clothes by Asian women found in our 1983 survey, reported above. It showed that an overwhelming majority of Pakistani (79 per cent) and Bangladeshi (85 per cent) women, almost all of them Muslims, always wore Asian clothes, compared with 43 per cent Indian and only 27 per cent African Asian women, as presented in Table 9.6.

Table 9.6 The wearing of Asian clothes (percentages)

Asian clothes worn	Indian		African Asian		Pakistani		Bangladeshi	
	Men	Women	Men	Women	Men	Women	Men	Women
Always	6	43	1	27	7	79	7	85
Sometimes	51	48	41	63	77	18	69	14
Never	43	8	58	10	16	3	24	0
16–34-year-olds								
Always	2	18	1	9	1	72	4	78
Sometimes	47	73	37	78	79	26	61	21
Never	52	8	62	13	20	2	34	1
All ages, if sometimes, then								
In own home	86	65	81	71	94	95	95	90
At social events	44	95	73	94	61	98	55	78

Source: SCPR/PSI Survey 1994 (Modood *et al.* 1997)

Young Asians (16–34-year-olds) also showed interesting ethnic differences, with an overwhelming majority of Pakistani and Bangladeshi young women showing a very high adherence to wearing Asian clothes all the time, but a very significant decline in the number of Indian and African Asian young women who always wore Asian clothes. Therefore, it is clear that ethnic differences between Asian groups would continue in the future, since they are mainly linked to religion, social class and origin.

It is relevant to mention here that Asian clothes are also getting popular in Britain, in that several fashion houses have been set up to meet the demands of this new trend. There are also many shops selling loose cloth and ready-made Asian clothes in areas of Asian settlement. In addition, a growing number of tailors now specialise in Asian clothes. Weddings and birthday parties as well as *Eid*, *Diwali* and *Basakhi* festivals are special occasions, when Asians, particularly women and children, like to wear new clothes. Therefore, a few weeks before such festivals, shops selling Asian clothes or loose cloth look very busy. In fact, some of the ceremonies which go with an Asian wedding in the subcontinent are now performed in almost exactly the same way in Britain. Similarly, the latest fashion in clothes and jewellery in the countries of origin are also copied, sometimes in modified form, in Britain. Asian press and broadcasting media and specialist magazines targeted at Asians help to publicise the latest trends in clothes and jewellery too. Asian fashion shows are organised for this purpose and sometimes are shown on Asian television programmes, such as Network East or the specialised cable television Channel Zee TV.

Chapter 10

Responses of policy makers and professionals

It is clear from the evidence presented in previous chapters that young Asians in Britain face two main types of difficulty. The first is the same type of prejudice and discrimination by some white people that first generation Asians have experienced and to a large extent tolerated. However, unlike their parents, it appears that young Asians are not prepared to accept hostility and discrimination as an inevitable part of living in Britain. The second is a social and psychological gap between young Asians and their parents due to a difference in social environment and education. The world at home is generally different from that of school and what they see in the media. However, young Asians are part of both worlds, which sometimes leads to tensions and conflict within Asian families. How far is this situation understood by professional and policy makers who run the institutions of society?

In 1977, a report by the CRC stated that 'the extent and type of differences between the needs of the urban deprived and the needs of ethnic minorities is the difference between "urban deprivation" and what has been called "racial disadvantage": that is, the disadvantages experienced by racial minorities which spring from racial prejudice, intolerance and less equal treatment in society' (CRC 1977). As part of the 1983 survey of parents and young people, professionals dealing with young people and local policy makers were also interviewed for nine local authority areas where parents and young people had been interviewed between 27 April and 4 August 1984. In this chapter, findings from those interviews are presented to show the awareness of the relevant policy makers and professionals of the problems of young Asians and other young people, and what solutions and remedies are suggested to deal with these problems. First, we look at the views of forty-four councillors, policy makers, who were either the chair or the vice-chair of employment, education, and youth and community services committees.

POLICY MAKERS

Most councillors felt that white and ethnic minority youth faced different problems; only nine of the forty-four councillors thought that they faced the same difficulties and disadvantages. The biggest difference was in finding jobs, followed by the experience of racial discrimination and the problems associated with having a different culture and lifestyle to the white majority. In the opinion of councillors, Afro-Caribbean young people were more likely to face difficulties in finding jobs, to experience racial discrimination and to have lack of family support. Asian young people, it was felt, were especially likely to face difficulties because of language and cultural differences. Table 10.1 shows the details of responses.

It appears from these responses that only three policy makers thought that Asian young people faced difficulties in finding jobs and only one showed awareness of their difficulties in education, compared with white young people. The majority of the councillors associated the difficulties young Asians faced with language

Table 10.1 'Ethnic minority and white youth face different disadvantages and difficulties'

	All councillors nos.	Difficulties facing ethnic minorities		
		All groups nos.	Asian nos.	Afro-Caribbean nos.
No difference	9	—	—	—
Finding job	21	18	3	8
Racial discrimination	16	13	6	6
Different culture and lifestyle	11	6	9	5
Language problem	7	5	8	1
Adjusting to British culture	7	2	8	2
Education	9	8	1	2
Lack of family support	3	1	2	6
Other	13	4	—	3
Size of sample	44	44	44	44

Source: 1984 survey

problems, culture, lifestyle and adjusting to British culture. However, when asked about the special needs of ethnic minority youth,
their views became clearer. The respondents thought that ethnic
minority youth had different needs in a number of different areas.
Education, careers advice and recreation were mentioned by more
than half of the policy makers, as shown in Table 10.2.

Table 10.2 Differing needs of ethnic minority and white youth

Needs different in	Councillors nos.
Education	31
Careers advice	27
Recreation	23
Training	12
Housing	11
Different employment prospects	35
Size of sample	44

Source: 1984 survey

The responses in Table 10.2 show that a significant majority of
councillors were aware of the different needs and different prospects of ethnic minority young people in finding jobs. The main
difference in employment prospects was thought to be that ethnic
minorities faced racial discrimination. Some councillors also mentioned the different job aspirations of white and ethnic minority
young people. When asked, forty-three of forty-four councillors
said their council had an equal opportunity policy but a majority
were unable to give details. However, two qualitative comments are
presented in this context regarding employment prospects:

> Employers still discriminate. The ethnic young people have to be
> treated the same as whites if they have the same qualifications.
> Employers are inclined to take on those young people with
> qualifications, as for example, store keepers but they pay them
> at a cheap rate. We would like to encourage equal opportunities.
>   (Chair of education committee)

> Their educational and language attainment is less than that for
> white youth and even when their attainment is equal to whites
> they are being discriminated against when applying for jobs –
> even in applying for council jobs there was an instance in which

someone was discriminated against. The council employs 3–4 per cent ethnic minorities but the proportion in the population is 17 per cent ethnic minority.

(Chair of education committee)

These comments show that some policy makers are aware of racial discrimination, even practised by their own councils. On the question of the special needs of ethnic minorities in education, thirty-one of the forty-four councillors interviewed believed that ethnic minority young people had different educational needs to whites. The main difference was thought to be in terms of language differences and other problems associated with belonging to a minority culture. Particularly for Asians, different cultural traditions, religious practices and recreational preferences were mentioned. In this context, a multi-cultural curriculum was generally cited as the best way for their different educational needs. Several councillors mentioned fears of a 'white backlash' if drastic changes were made. One councillor explained:

Differences in culture spill over into education. Whites cope better and get better results in tests. I have seen this in my job as well as a councillor. It is to do with Asian culture and home background. It's not the school education which causes the poor results. It is the cultural background. They go home and speak their language, that is the problem, it is what is behind the spoken and written word that they don't grasp and this is something very difficult to touch. Problems can only be resolved through time.

(Chair of education committee)

Another commented:

Quite a lot of our schools are predominantly coloured so we fronted a campaign for policies to cater for their needs. Section 11 money from the Government [for the particular needs of local ethnic minority populations] has been used to provide extra staff in these schools and a number of teachers from ethnic minorities have been employed. Multi-cultural awareness is introduced in teaching.

(Vice-chair of education committee)

It is interesting to note from the first comment that the whole blame for the poor results of Asians in examinations was placed

on their cultural background and mother tongue. There is no
research evidence which supports such stereotypical views. If the
chair of an education committee believes in these views, then what
sorts of policy and practice should be expected from the relevant
council to meet the special needs of Asians and other ethnic minority young people in education?

The majority of councillors, twenty-seven out of forty-four,
believed that ethnic minority young people differed from whites
in one main respect: as far as need for careers advice was concerned. In the first instance, many ethnic minorities and Asians in
particular were thought to have 'too high' job aspirations (see
Chapter 4). Other differences included help in overcoming racial
prejudice of employers and help in countering family pressures to
go in for a limited range of options. The majority of councillors
admitted that they had not taken any action or were planning to
implement new policies to meet these differing needs.

It is interesting to note that only a quarter of the councillors
interviewed thought that ethnic minority youth had different training needs to whites. This is despite the very high unemployment
among ethnic minority young people. Councillors thought that
ethnic minority youth needed special help because of cultural and
language difficulties and also in dealing with racial prejudice. When
asked whether any action had been taken to deal with the special
needs, only a small number of councils had started special training
initiatives, e.g. courses to improve English, and self-help funding of
projects and training workshops. Three qualitative comments will
help to show the reasons for some of the answers on special training for ethnic minority young people:

> Because of cultural and language difficulties they are starting
> from a lower level even if they reached the same standard at
> school. They don't interview as well.
>
> (Vice-chair of education committee)

> Special entry courses for under-achieving coloured youngsters to
> get to college without A-levels, find the need is for more quali-
> fications but try to make up for under-achievers.
>
> (Chair of education committee)

> There are grants from the unemployment subcommittee to the
> racial minority associations, where a kind of training takes
> place for unemployed young people. Try not to distinguish by

having courses especially for certain groups but some courses do have more ethnics attending them and extra funds go to them.

(Vice-chair of education committee)

What is clear from some of the responses is that policy makers were obsessed with the cultural and language differences of Asians and saw them as causes for most of the difficulties Asian young people faced in education, careers advice and training, although the reality is quite different and although these views are almost opposite to the ones on these aspects expressed by young Asians and Asian parents (see Chapters 3 and 4). Policy makers to some extent accepted that there were different needs of young Asians and other ethnic minorities, but little was done to meet their needs. It is worth pointing out that some of the language used in their responses, such as 'coloured youngsters', is outdated, which also shows that the councillors' knowledge about more recent developments is limited.

In the field of recreation, twenty-three out of the forty-four councillors believed that Asian and other ethnic minority youth had different recreational needs to their white counterparts. Differences in sporting and cultural preferences were mentioned, as was the need for separate recreational facilities for Muslim girls. One councillor commented:

It is all to do with females and their cultural background e.g. swimming. They have to be allowed separate lessons and special clothing. It is difficult because we would like to integrate rather than separate but it's impossible due to female cultural problems.

(Vice-chair of education committee)

How was the need of Asian young people assessed? Seventeen out of the forty-four councillors did not know how it was done. Some mentioned that need assessment was usually done by informal reports from liaison officers, community groups and youth workers. One councillor explained:

We have a specialist liaison officer who reports to council committees (for needs of all young people) and a special advisor to the directorate of education on Asian young people.

(Vice-chair of education, youth and community services committee)

Another councillor, chair of an education committee, said that they assessed the needs of Asian young people 'just through the multi-cultural education support group'. It is interesting to point out that almost half of the councillors interviewed (twenty) did not know how many youth workers were employed by their council specially to deal with the problems of ethnic minority youth. The majority of the rest (eleven councillors) thought their councils employed fifteen or more of these youth workers. It was also believed that some of these youth workers were allocated to Asian and other ethnic minority groups, but most councillors were not sure of the exact numbers involved.

If councils were not meeting the needs of Asian and other ethnic minority young people in a satisfactory way, then what support was being provided for ethnic minority self-help groups? The majority of councillors said that it was their council policy to give assistance to ethnic minority self-help groups. This was mainly in the form of financial and administrative help, and of help with accommodation for ethnic minority groups. Some of these groups were mainly Asian, mainly Afro-Caribbean, mainly white or multi-racial. We asked councillors to tell us the nature of and target groups for special projects or centres for ethnic minority young people. Details are presented in Table 10.3.

Table 10.3 Projects or centres for ethnic minority youth

	All groups	Afro-Caribbean	Asian	Other ethnic minority
Employment	14	3	3	3
Training	29	4	5	—
Education	11	7	5	1
Housing	2	1	—	—

It is clear from Table 10.3 that most of the projects and centres were for all ethnic groups, including whites, and a few were specifically for Asians, Afro-Caribbeans and other ethnic minority groups. This shows that the council's policy was for more integrated projects rather than separate ethnicity-based activities.

Almost all the councillors interviewed (forty-three out of forty-four) claimed that their council had an equal opportunity policy, and forty-one of them also claimed that their council encouraged other employers in the area to adopt equal opportunity policies.

When asked whether they sent staff on relevant training, twenty-five councillors claimed that it was council policy. Most of these courses lasted less than a week. Therefore, it appears that local councils, like other large employers, had equal opportunity policies but very little was being done to implement them. In this context, councillors were asked 'What needs to be done to meet the needs of a multi-cultural, multi-racial society?' Many councillors believed that changing attitudes through education in the broader sense was the main thing which could be done in their area to meet these needs. Other things mentioned by a few councillors were more jobs and better recreational facilities for ethnic minorities. However, it is interesting to point out that only a minority of the policy makers thought that enough had been done already. Some illustrative comments on changing attitudes include:

> Education, a long slow process. An awareness that other people's traditions and values are not less than yours. Most people are passively discriminating.
>
> (Chair of education committee)

> The main thing is a need to change attitudes in the community and even on the council. This can't be done by a council – it can only be done by evolutionary process. The mistake we have made in this area is that we have tried to force things in order to create a multi-racial society and what we have created is a backlash.
>
> (Chair of youth employment committee)

It is clear from the above comments that the attitudes of white people needed to be changed as part of an educational process and not through telling people what to do. Persuasion needs to be a priority. However, some councillors had also mentioned the other side of the coin, that is, to adapt services to meet the socio-cultural needs of ethnic minorities. A few examples of responses from councillors on this will help to illustrate this dimension:

> More of an identification of the needs of ethnic minorities, and that would bring to our attention the need to direct resources to them.
>
> (Chair of employment committee)

> Given space, buildings, etc., so they [ethnic minorities] can organise and they can determine what they want and need and

a proper mechanism so their voice will be heard and notice taken.

(Vice-chair of youth employment committee)

More explicit equal opportunity policy and every policy of the council should have racial awareness to see if the policies meet the need of the ethnic minorities.

(Chair of education committee)

One of the objectives of the survey among policy makers was to look at examples of good and bad practice among councils, by looking at council practices, area by area, which were relevant to young people. The most significant finding was that there was little agreement between councillors on what the procedures and policies in their councils were. Thus the prevalence of good and bad council practice was difficult to assess. However, some relevant findings and comments are used below to analyse the situation.

In seven councils out of eight, there was unanimous agreement on whether there was a committee which co-ordinated policy on young people. However, in fact, only two councils had such a committee. Similarly, in only three councils out of eight was there agreement as to whether any particular department had been given specific responsibility for youth policy matters. Two councils had such a department and one did not. Estimates of the number of youth workers employed specifically to deal with the problems of ethnic minority young people varied widely between councillors in all councils. Although councillors in seven out of eight councils were agreed that it was council policy to give assistance to ethnic minority self-help groups, in only one area was there agreement on how many groups had been helped in the past years or the type of help which had been given. In only one council were councillors agreed as to whether the council had set up any projects or centres designed primarily for Asian and other ethnic minority youth. In fact, even this council had not set up any projects specifically for ethnic minority youth. Therefore, what emerges from chairs and vice-chairs of various committees is their lack of full knowledge about the policies and procedures of their own councils relevant to Asian and other ethnic minority young people in their areas. If they themselves were not sure, then what expectations do they have about meeting the needs of their multi-racial, multi-cultural constituents? Also, what knowledge, practices and attitudes do relevant professionals have to meet the needs of their multi-racial and multi-cultural clients?

PROFESSIONALS

It appears that the professionals often saw the problems of young Asians only in terms of their own specialised profession. Social workers, for example, saw physical living conditions or low income as the causes of problems. Housing managers recognised the need for bigger houses for Asian extended families. School teachers related the problems of young Asians to lack of competence in English. However, some well-informed professionals, such as community workers, saw the specific issues of cultural differences and contrast compounded by racial prejudice and discrimination. The situation of young Asians was a product of both, and their responses were to the combined effects of both. Both these factors can result in conflict, not only with parents, but also with the institutions of society. One recent example of this conflict was the disturbances in Bradford (June 1995) in which young Asians were involved. The disturbances started over the treatment of Asian women by the police and later developed into a protest not only against the police, but also against discrimination against Asian young people in getting jobs, non-representation and lack of equal opportunity policies. There were also signs that young Asians were not happy about their parents' tolerance of racial prejudice and discrimination, and this showed the generation gap. Authority was resented and the pleas of older Asian leaders and parents were largely ignored in the initial stages of the protest. The same pattern has been repeated in other areas such as Birmingham, Luton and Manchester, where young Asians, humiliated by being treated as 'second-class' citizens, had revolted against this treatment and sometimes against their own community leaders who appeared to accept it (for attitudes to community organisations, see Chapter 11).

Since education has appeared as a key area in terms of providing equality of opportunity for young Asians and also of helping to change attitudes towards a multi-cultural society, we examined the attitudes of teachers in this context in Chapter 3. What they showed, on the one hand, was that teachers on the whole had stereotypical views of Asian young people. These views related to their competence in English, performance in public examinations, and lack of Asian parents' involvement in the education of their children and in extra-curricular activities in schools. On the other hand, multi-cultural education was seen as something marginal and not very significant. What this means is that there is a mismatch between the views of policy makers, who saw education playing an important role in a multi-racial, multi-cultural Britain, and professional teachers, who saw the role of education as marginal in changing attitudes. Therefore, it appears that more needs to be done to monitor the policy and its practice by professionals, if we want to see some results in terms of equal opportunities and facilitating the effective representation and integration of young British Asians in society.

Chapter 11

Community responses and political participation

COMMUNITY RESPONSES

Asian communities differ greatly in the help they offer to their
members. Generally, they offer basic welfare services, through
their close family networks or through their community organisations. But they are unable to cope with the more subtle problems
faced by young Asians and Asian communities. There is a common
myth among white policy makers and professionals that, due to the
close family system, Asians do not have any problems and that
their needs are met within their own communities. While it is true
that the extended kinship group does meet some basic needs, there
is little evidence that Asian millionaires take much interest in
providing community welfare facilities on the Jewish communities'
pattern.

Asian leaders and organisations are generally thought to play an
important role in the life of their communities. There have been
several developments in terms of the nature and activities of Asian
organisations. These include social, welfare, religious, women's,
professional and political groups. Some cover a combination of
these interests. They include 'formal' and 'traditional' leaders
(Anwar 1991a). Formal leaders are those who represent Asian
communities through their organisations, whether elected, nomi-
nated or self-appointed. They are mainly educated, and are professionals who have contacts with the wider society. Their role is
important in inter-ethnic situations, where they are often seen as
representatives of their communities. The traditional leaders on the
other hand draw their support from kinship or religious groups.
Their leadership depends on age, length of stay in Britain, number
of relatives living in an area and religious position. The traditional

leaders normally play their part in intra-ethnic situations, because sometimes they are more effective in mobilising support, particularly on religious issues or issues relevant to the country of origin.

It is estimated that there are almost 1,800 Asian organisations throughout Britain. These include local, regional and national organisations. They are mainly based on ethnic, regional or national origin or on religion, although some are professional ones, e.g. the Overseas Doctors' Association (ODA). The role of Asian organisations and Asian leaders in Britain is crucial as they provide the channels of communication with the wider society's institutions. Some well-established national Asian organisations include: the Confederation of Indian Organisations, the Standing Conference of Pakistani Organisations, and the Federation of Bangladeshi Organisations. There are also several national Asian religious organisations, which include the Union of Muslim Organisations (UMO), the UK Islamic Mission, the Supreme Council of Sikhs, and several Hindu organisations.

How are such organisations viewed by Asians? We asked respondents in the 1975 and 1983 surveys how far they thought the Asian organisations recognised and met the needs of young Asians. It appeared that attitudes towards Asian organisations had become more positive over time. In 1975, half of the young Asians in the sample were critical of Asian organisations' not recognising the needs of young Asians, but in 1983, only one in three young Asians were critical, as shown in Tables 11.1 and 11.2.

There seemed to be a proportionately more positive change in the attitudes of Asian parents between 1975 and 1983. Young Asians' views in 1983 were also the opposite of those found in 1975. This suggests that Asian organisations may increasingly be

Table 11.1 'Asian organisations do not recognise the needs of young Asians'

Response	Asian parents		Young people	
	1975 %	1983 %	1975 %	1983 %
Agree	32	50	20	48
Neither agree nor disagree	22	24	28	24
Disagree	42	26	44	28
Size of sample	570	1,117	212	944

Table 11.2 'Asian organisations do not do much to help the problems of young Asians'

	Asian parents		Young people	
Response	1975 %	1983 %	1975 %	1983 %
Agree	35	52	16	51
Neither agree nor disagree	14	20	31	21
Disagree	45	28	50	28
Size of sample	570	1,117	212	944

more responsive to the needs and problems faced by young Asians. Some positive and negative qualitative comments will be useful to illustrate the general thrust:

They provide good facilities like sports facilities and outings.

(Young Asian)

They [organisations] try to help, for example, solve the problems of unemployment, but it is up to the authorities to try and help us as well.

(Asian parent)

They do not let us have a say. And do not give us a chance to show how we feel.

(Young Asian)

They are too involved in internal politics and fighting amongst themselves.

(Young Asian)

In the 1990s, it appears that several national, regional and local organisations have been started by young Asians to meet the needs of young people. Such organisations relate to art and culture but also include some professional organisations, such as the Kashmiri and Pakistani Professionals' Association. Some of these associations are not only used to draw the attention of the relevant institutions of society to the particular problems of Asian young people but also provide a network for the mobilisation of their members on certain issues relevant to their communities. The new generation of Asian professionals is well equipped to make demands for equality of treatment and to highlight racial discrimination, because of their education and working in Britain.

Some young Asians are also participating in mainstream organi-sations, including political parties. This development is happening at a time when the first generation Asian leaders have achieved a modest representation at local and national levels as elected, appointed or co-opted members. However, young Asians feel that political parties in Britain need to do more to provide equal access to Asians and other ethnic minorities, as is reflected in the follow-ing comment:

> We need to stress and remind the British political parties that second generation Asians do not need patronage, like our fathers, in the political system, we would like our share of representation. If some political parties are not prepared to treat us equally we want to campaign against them and mobilise support to defeat their candidates at selection and elections. We have all the skills to represent. No more excuses are accep-table.
>
> (Young Asian, interviewed April 1994, during local election campaign)

The views of young Asians on representation are clear from this comment. Therefore, we now examine the participation and repre-sentation of Asians in the British political system.

POLITICAL PARTICIPATION

It was pointed out in Chapter 2 that Asians are concentrated in some inner-city areas of Britain. This has implications for their participa-tion in the British political process. Their concentration in particular conurbations means that, at least in statistical terms, Asians are in a position to influence the vote in those areas. They are even further concentrated in some parliamentary constituencies and local elec-tion wards, and are therefore in a position to make an impact in those areas. The 1991 Census showed that there were seventy-eight parliamentary constituencies with more than 15 per cent ethnic minority population (twenty-three with over 30 per cent), and the majority were of Asian origin. In 1981, there were fifty-eight con-stituencies with more than 15 per cent of the total population living in households with the head born in the New Commonwealth and Pakistan (NCWP). It is estimated that, in 1997, there are more than seventy-five parliamentary constituencies with a 10 per cent Asian population. Birmingham Small Heath constituency has an Asian population of almost 50 per cent, followed by Ealing Southall with a similar percentage. There are also now several hundred local election wards with an Asian population, of 10 per cent, and more. The highest Asian population, of about 90 per cent, was recorded in Northcote ward in the London Borough of Ealing, followed by Spinney Hill in Leicester with an Asian population of about 80 per cent. However, it must be stressed here that it is not only the number of Asians in certain areas which makes those people electorally important but also whether they actively take part in the political process through registration on the electoral register, and, if they are on the register, whether they come out to vote and how they compare with non-Asians in terms of such participation. We also need to look at how their representation at local and national levels compares with their numbers in the population. But first we will make some general historically relevant points.

Because of the historical and colonial links of Asians with Britain, they have a legal right to participate fully in the country's politics. This includes the right to vote and to be a candidate in local, national and European parliamentary elections. Such participation is not new. Three MPs from the Indian subcontinent were elected to the House of Commons before World War II. The first, Dadabhai Naoroji, was elected over 100 years ago in 1892 as a Liberal, with a majority of five, at Finsbury Central. The second, Sir Mancherjee Bhownagree, was twice elected as a Conservative for Bethnal Green North East in 1895 and 1900. The third, Shapurji Saklatvala, was also twice elected for Battersea North, as a Labour candidate in 1922 and as a Communist in 1924. All three were Parsees. In the House of Lords, there was one member from the Indian subcontinent, Lord Sinha of Raipur (1863–1928). There are, at present, five Asian members of the House of Lords: Lords Chitnis, Desai, Paul and Bagri and Lady Flather, the first ethnic minority woman to join the House. At a local level, in 1934, Chunilal Katial, a medical doctor, was elected as a Labour councillor in Finsbury, north London, and, in 1938, he became the first Asian mayor in Britain. Krishna Menon, a teacher, was also elected in 1934 as a Labour councillor for St Pancras ward in London. During this period, in 1936, another doctor, Jainti Saggar, was also elected as a Labour councillor in Dundee and served for eighteen years. There are other examples too of Asians who were elected by their mainly white electorate, and of Asian women participating in many suffragette organisations at the beginning of this century. For example, Sophia Duleep Singh who lived in London, was a very active participant in the 1910s.

After World War II, due to the mass migration of Asians into Britain, in many areas the electorate became multi-racial, and it is in this context that we now examine the impact of Asians upon British politics. First, we examine registration, which is a fundamental prerequisite for participation in politics.

In the 1960s, it was found that less than half of all Commonwealth immigrants, including Asians, were registered (Deakin 1965). After a decade, a sample survey in 1974 of 227 Asians and Afro-Caribbeans and 175 whites showed that, although improvements had taken place, ethnic minorities were still five times as likely not to have registered to vote as whites (Anwar and Kohler 1975). It was found that 6 per cent of whites, compared with 27 per cent of Asians and 37 per cent of Afro-Caribbeans, were not registered. However, further research in two areas, Birmingham and Bradford, where fieldwork had been undertaken in 1974, showed a great improvement in the registration levels of Asians. In Birmingham, it was found that 5 per cent of Asians and 13 per cent of Afro-Caribbeans were not on the electoral register, compared with 4 per cent of whites. In Bradford, 9 per cent of Asians were not registered, as against 5 per cent of whites from the same areas (Anwar 1979). It appeared that this improvement took place because of the efforts of the then CRC, the two local authorities, local community relations councils, political parties and also some ethnic minority community groups. The ethnic minority press played an important role.

A survey in twenty-four parliamentary constituencies in 1979 showed that 23 per cent of Asians and 7 per cent of whites were not registered (Anwar 1980). Another survey in 1981 showed that in Inner London, Asians had double the non-registration rate of white people (27 per cent and 12 per cent respectively) (Todd and Butcher 1982). In 1983, a survey showed that 21 per cent of Asians but also 19 per cent of whites from the same areas were not registered (Anwar 1984). The fieldwork for the survey was undertaken in inner-city wards, where registration levels are generally low, and there were wide area variations. These variations were due to the policies of the local electoral registration officers (EROs) and the efforts of other concerned. A more recent national study of registration still showed the gaps between whites, Asians and blacks. It showed that 15 per cent of Asians, 24 per cent of blacks and only 6 per cent of whites were not registered (Smith 1993).

What are the reasons for non-registration? My research in the last twenty-four years has shown that, in addition to doubts about eligibility criteria, some Asians face language difficulty, general alienation from politics, and fear of racial harassment and racial attacks from the extreme right-wing groups who could identify Asian names on the register. The lack of relevant policies in the Registration Offices and political parties are also contributory factors to the non-registration of Asians.

If Asians are on the Register, do they come out to vote? Monitoring of various local and general elections in the last twenty years has shown that, on average, the Asian turn-out is generally higher than that of non-Asians from the same areas. For example, at the October 1974 general election, a survey in Bradford and Rochdale showed that the turn-out among Asians was 57.7 per cent, compared with 54.6 per cent for non-Asians (Anwar 1980). At the 1979 general election, Asian turn-out rates in 18 of the 19 constituencies monitored were higher than non-Asian. On average, it was 65 per cent for Asians and 61 per cent for non-Asians. In 1983, once again, we found that the Asian turn-out was higher than that of non-Asians. Overall the turn-out was 81 per cent for Asians and 60 per cent for non-Asians (Anwar 1984). A survey at the 1987 general election and another in 1991, before the 1992 general election, also showed that there was a greater likelihood of Asians turning out to vote (*Asian Times*, 5–11 June 1989; Amin and Richardson 1992). A similar pattern of higher turn-out of Asians was discovered in various surveys undertaken at local elections (Le Lohe 1975, 1984; Anwar 1986, 1994). Therefore, the greater likelihood of an Asian turn-out to vote suggests that Asians are capable of being more reliable voters and, consequently, in a better position to influence the outcome of elections in their areas of concentration.

It is worth pointing out here that, due to an increased political awareness among Asians generally and young Asians in particular, their membership of political parties has increased significantly in the last few years. In some areas like Birmingham, Bradford, Leicester, Southall and Tower Hamlets, Asians are now dominating the local political party associations, particularly in the Labour Party, and in some cases they are being accused of 'taking over'. This has led to problems of membership and selection of candidates in some areas. The Labour Party National Executive Committee (NEC) had to intervene several times in the selection of both white and Asian candidates. The signs are that, with young Asians taking increasing interest in the political process, the membership of political parties and attendance at political party meetings is likely to increase in the next few years.

The voting patterns of Asians, compared with those of whites and Afro-Caribbeans, are examined, briefly here to show how the former are changing over time and in particular due to the emergence of second generation Asian electors. At the 1979 general election, an exit poll in twenty-four parliamentary constituencies revealed that 86 per cent of Asians, 90 per cent of Afro-Caribbeans and 50 per cent of whites voted for the Labour Party (Anwar 1980). However, in some constituencies like Rochdale, up to 50 per cent of Asians voted for the Liberal Party candidate, and in some other constituencies over 15 per cent of Asians voted for the Conservative Party. At the 1983 general election, a national exit poll showed that the majority of ethnic minorities had voted Labour (57 per cent) but 24 per cent and 16 per cent had voted Conservative and Alliance respectively (Anwar 1986). However, it appeared that the solid support for Labour among Afro-Caribbean voters remained while Asians were slowly moving towards other parties as well. For example, in Bristol East, with a mainly Afro-Caribbean population, there was recorded the highest ethnic minority vote (93 per cent) for the Labour Party; for the Conservatives the highest was in Croydon North East (27 per cent) and for the Alliance in Rochdale (54 per cent), the last two with a predominantly Asian electorate. This trend of support continued. At the 1987 general election, 66.8 per cent Asians intended to vote for the Labour Party, 22.7 per cent for the Conservative Party and 10 per cent for the Alliance (*Asian Times*, May 1987). An exit poll confirmed this pattern, showing that 61 per cent of Asians had voted for Labour, compared with 20 per cent for Conservatives and 17 per cent for the Alliance. Once again, there were area variations. Decrease in Labour Party support among Asians was also shown in a survey carried out by National Opinion Polls (NOP) before the 1992 general election. It showed that 55 per cent of Asians intended to vote for the Labour Party and, while 18 per cent of respondents were still undecided, the others were likely to vote for the Conservatives and Liberal Democrats.

These voting patterns over time show that the majority of Asians still vote for the Labour Party but a significant minority vote for the Conservative Party or for the Liberal Democrats, and this trend is likely to continue in the near future. One reason for this is that the Labour Party is still perceived as more sympathetic to Asians and other ethnic minorities and 'supports the working class'. This pattern is also found in the United States, where the Democratic Party has always received the majority of black votes due to a similar perception (Cavanagh 1984). In addition, personal involvement with Asians and the popularity of the respective candidates from these parties has been one of the important factors in attracting the Asian vote, as was demonstrated by Cyril Smith in Rochdale (Anwar 1973, 1975). It also appears that the efforts of the Conservative Party to win support amongst Asians is making a significant difference. The values of Asian communities – home ownership and emphasis on family life – and their educational and occupational trends, are believed to be more relevant to the Conservative Party philosophy. These factors and the efforts of the Conservative Central Office (see below) are bringing more Asians, particularly young professionals and business persons, to join and support the Conservative Party. This trend is similar to that of the Jewish community in Britain, which also shifted its support, over time, from the Labour Party to the Conservative Party (Alderman 1983, 1993). However, it appears that the policies of the political parties, their regular contacts with Asians, Asians' membership of political parties, the organisation and mobilisation of Asians at local and national levels (sometimes through their own organisations), the candidates', personal contact and familiarity with Asians, and presence of Asian candidates in elections are important factors in attracting electoral support from Asians in Britain.

As stated above, the policies and initiatives taken by the political parties to encourage Asian participation in the British political process are important. It is clear that, more recently, the leaders of major political parties have openly sought Asian support without the fear of losing white voters. Some political parties have special set-ups to attract Asian and other ethnic minority support. The Conservative Party has had an Ethnic Minority Unit in the Conservative Central Office's Department of Community Affairs since 1976. Its objective is to make party members aware of the growing importance of Asians and other ethnic minority electors, to influence party policy to improve the image of the party among Asians and other ethnic minorities, and, as a result, to seek their support. The Unit helped form an Anglo-Asian Conservative Society through which it recruited Asians directly into the party. At the last count, it had about thirty local branches. This development was followed by the formation of the Anglo-West Indian Conservative Society with the same objective. More recently, these societies have been replaced by a national organisation, the One Nation Forum, with similar objectives, but the Anglo-Asian and Anglo-West Indian Societies continue their activities at local level. Many young Asians, both at national and local levels, are members. They get involved in election campaigns as Conservative Party workers, and several are coming forward as party candidates. It is relevant to mention here that John Major hosted a dinner for Asian multi-millionaires at 10 Downing Street on the first anniversary of his becoming the Conservative Party leader, as part of a campaign to build bridges with the Asians (Anwar 1994). In 1993, he said to a meeting of 800 Asians, 'we want you in the Conservative Party – there must be no barriers' (*Sunday Telegraph*, 18 April 1993). In January 1997, Major's visit to the Indian subcontinent was also seen partly as an attempt to win electoral support from Asians in Britain, and this was discussed in the media widely. After his trip, Major made a speech at the Commonwealth Institute. He also personally appeared at a gathering of his party's One Nation Forum on 18 January. Michael Howard, the Home Secretary, in a recent speech (6 February 1997), also voiced his appreciation of the role of Asians in the prosperity of Britain and reiterated that Asian values were closer to the philosophy of the Conservative Party. He said that, therefore, Asians were natural Conservative Party supporters. All these activities show that the Conservative Party is using various methods to attract support among Asians.

The Labour Party Race and Action Group (LPRAG) was set up in 1975, as a pressure group to educate and advise the party on relevant issues. Then there was a long campaign to set up Black Sections in the Labour Party (Shukra 1990; Jeffers 1991). This issue was debated and defeated at several Labour Party annual conferences in the 1980s. Finally, as a result of various discussions, the Labour Party NEC set up a Black and Asian Advisory Committee, followed by a Black Socialist Society, similar to the Party's women's and local government committees. The objective of the Society is primarily to get and maintain ethnic minorities' support for the party. An officer is also appointed at the Labour Party national headquarters to deal with ethnic minorities. More recently, the Labour Party agreed a policy on the Kashmir issue after a lot of pressure from the Pakistani and Kashmiri supporters of the Labour Party, including Labour councillors (Labour Party

Debates, September 1995). The Labour Party Leader, Tony Blair, met the then Pakistani Prime Minister, Benazir Bhutto, in October 1995, when she stopped for few hours in London, on her way to the United States. It is understood he was the only leading British politician to see her and she also thanked him for the Labour Party's recently approved policy regarding Kashmir. It is also worth mentioning here that, after the 1995 Labour Party Conference, there was a campaign by Pakistanis and Kashmiris to get a similar policy approved at the Conservative Party Conference. However, there was not enough time to organise such a campaign properly, and the role of the Conservative Party Annual Conference, unlike the Labour Party's, is advisory and not policy making. The Labour leader, with his wife, visited the Regent's Park Mosque in London on Saturday 8 February 1997 when the Muslim community celebrated *Eid ul fitr*. Some saw this as an early initiative by the Labour Party leader directed at the Muslims, ahead of the 1997 general election. It appears from various other developments, monitored by the author, that up to the next general election both the political parties are likely to compete for the Asian communities' support. This does not mean that the Liberal Democrats and even the Scottish National Party (SNP) are not in this race.

The Liberal Party used to have a Community Relations Panel in the 1970s, which included ethnic minority members. It met regularly to discuss relevant issues and formulated not only policies to attract ethnic minority members, but also campaigning strategies at elections specially directed at them. It appears that now the Liberal Democrats are following a similar arrangement. More recently, the Liberal Democrats' leader personally took an interest in this connection. In June 1991, a special organisation with the name of 'Asian Liberal Democrats' was formed to attract Asian support for the Party. An Asian was also a member of the Liberal Democrats National Executive. Like the leader of the Conservative Party, the leader of the Liberal Democrats has held important meetings with Asian businessmen and others to attract financial, as well as electoral support, for the party, among Asians. It appears that the party is having some success in this context.

The SNP is also trying to examine ways of getting Asians to support the party and some Asian candidates contesting seats for the party at the 1997 general election.

One way to examine the response of the political parties to the participation of Asians in politics is to look at the number of Asian

candidates adopted by the parties in the last few general elections
and the representation of Asians at national and local levels. The
first Asian candidate put forward by a major political party after
1945 was Sardar K.S.N. Ahluwala, who contested Willesden West
for the Liberal Party in 1950. At the February 1974 election, the
Labour Party put forward an Asian from Glasgow to contest East
Fife, and the Liberal Party selected one Asian for Coventry South
East. There were no Asian candidates selected by the main political
parties at the October 1974 general election. However, things
improved at the 1979 general election, when, out of the five ethnic
minority candidates put forward by the three main political parties,
three were Asians (seven others stood for the minor parties). Two
Asians were selected by the Conservative Party and one by the
Liberal Party. This was the first time since 1945 that the Conservative Party had selected ethnic minority candidates. In the event, all
the Asians lost, and this applied to all the other ethnic minority
candidates – because they contested seats where there was no chance
of winning, irrespective of the political party. At the 1983 general
election, two-thirds of the eighteen ethnic minority candidates who
stood for the major political parties were Asians. However, as in
1979, no Asian candidate contested a winnable or safe seat. The
main political parties nevertheless continued to attract Asian electoral support, and selected eighteen Asian candidates at the 1987
general election, out of a total of twenty-seven ethnic minority
candidates. Only one of them, Keith Vaz (Leicester East), was
returned – for the Labour Party. One other Asian, Mohammad
Aslam (Nottingham East), the Labour Party candidate, lost the
seat only by 456 votes, because of divided Labour Party support
due to a dispute about his selection. Three Afro-Caribbean Labour
MPs were also returned at this election: Paul Boateng (Brent South),
Diane Abbott (Hackney North and Stoke Newington) and Bernie
Grant (Tottenham). The three London MPs were all elected in safe
Labour seats. However, Keith Vaz won his seat with a swing of over
9 per cent from the Conservative candidate. As far as the general
performance of Asian candidates was concerned, it was like that of
other party candidates in the same regions. That election provided
further evidence that Asians and other ethnic minority candidates
were not vote losers any longer and, in some cases, they were in fact
improving the party position by attracting more voters.

One clear indication of the acceptance of Asian candidates by
white electors came from the Langbaurgh parliamentary by-elec-

tion in November 1991, in an area which had only 0.7 per cent of ethnic minorities. Dr Ashok Kumar gained this seat for Labour from the Conservative Party with a swing of 3.6 per cent. This increased the number of Asian MPs to two until the 1992 general election. At that election, out of the twenty-three ethnic minority candidates selected by the main political parties, sixteen were of Asian origin, as shown in Table 11.3. Out of the twenty-two constituencies contested by ethnic minority candidates, six had very small ethnic minority populations, less than the national average of 5.5 per cent. This also showed that political parties were now prepared to put forward Asians and other ethnic minority candidates in 'snow-white' areas. On the other hand, Asians do not hesitate to stand against each other. In one constituency, Ealing Southall, in 1992, two Asian candidates stood against each other, one for the Labour Party and the other for the Liberal Democrats. The sixteen Asian candidates included four Labour, six Conservatives and six Liberal Democrats. Table 11.3 also shows the details of their constituencies and their respective parties, ethnic minority population in 1991, and the political parties' majorities at the 1987 and 1992 general elections. In addition to one Asian sitting Labour MP (elected in 1987), another Asian, Piara Khabra (Ealing Southall), was elected. At the same time, the first Asian in recent times, Nirj Deva (Brentford and Isleworth), was elected to represent the Conservative Party in the House of Commons. However, Dr Kumar (Langbaurgh) lost his seat, which he had won in the by-election, by a small margin to the Conservative candidate.

A close examination of the election results shows that, overall, the performance of Asian candidates, which included several young Asians, was better in some areas than others. The negative swing for Asian candidates, for example, for a particular political party was fairly similar to the other political party candidates' in the region. In one case, against the regional trend, one Asian Conservative candidate, Abdul Qayyum Chaudhary (Birmingham Small Heath), produced a swing of 2.5 per cent to the Conservatives, whereas generally in Birmingham, the swing was on average 2.6 per cent to Labour. This constituency has a 40 per cent Asian population and the controversial selection of a Labour white candidate could have contributed to this swing.

At the 1992 general election, a lot of media interest was shown in the newly formed Islamic Party of Britain. The impression given by

Table 11.3 Asian candidates representing main political parties, 1992 general election

Party	Candidate	Constituency	Ethnic minority populations, 1991 %	Majority at 1987 %	Majority at 1992 %
Lab.	Claude Moraes	Harrow West	22.5	Cons. 25.0	Cons. 32.7
Lab.	Piara Khabra	Ealing Southall	51.2	Lab. 15.3	Lab. 13.9
Lab.	Ashok Kumar*	Langbaurgh	0.7	Cons. 3.3	Cons. 2.4
Lab.	Keith Vaz	Leicester East	38.0	Lab. 3.7	Lab. 22.8
Cons.	Abdul Q. Chaudhary	Birmingham Small Heath	55.0	Lab. 35.2	Lab. 39.2
Cons.	Nirj J. Deva	Brentford and Isleworth	18.4	Cons. 14.5	Cons. 3.9
Cons.	Mohammed Khamisa	Birmingham Sparkbrook	49.0	Lab. 45.2	Lab. 40.2
Cons.	Mohammad Riaz	Bradford North	20.7	Lab. 3.3	Lab. 15.7
Cons.	Mohammad Rizvi	Edinburgh Leith		Lab. 26.5	Lab. 12.4
Cons.	Andrew Popat	Bradford South	8.0	Lab. 0.6	Lab. 9.3
Lib.D.	Mohammad A. Ali	Liverpool Riverside	12.5	Lab. 59.4	Lab. 64.4
Lib.D.	Zerbanoo Gifford	Hertsmere	4.6	Cons. 32.8	Cons. 33.1
Lib.D.	Pash Nandhra	Ealing Southall	51.2	Lab. 15.3	Lab. 13.9
Lib.D.	Vinod Sharma	Halesowen and Stourbridge	3.6	Cons 22.3	Cons 15.0
Lib.D.	Marcello Verma	Cynon Valley	0.7	Lab. 56.7	Lab. 56.2
Lib.D.	Peter Veruna	Cardiff South and Penarth	6.4	Lab. 10.2	Lab. 21.9

Sources: 1987 and 1992 general election results; 1991 Census of Population, produced by NEMDA, January 1994
*In the 1991 by-election Dr Kumar's (Lab.) majority was 3.8 per cent.

the media was that the candidates of the Islamic Party, led by white converts, might receive significant support from the Muslim electors. The party contested only four parliamentary seats, three in Bradford, which has a significant number of Muslim electors, and one in London (Streatham). All four candidates performed poorly. On average they received 0.6 per cent of the votes cast in the four constituencies. Their performance, and the poor result of independent and minor parties' candidates, support the author's earlier conclusions that such candidates, outside the main political parties, do not stand a chance of winning in the British electoral system (Anwar 1986).

At the time of writing, twenty-six Asian-origin candidates had been selected by the three main political parties. The SNP had also selected one Asian candidate in Glasgow, and the Referendum Party had selected six Asian candidates, five in London, for the 1997 election. Three important selections for the Labour Party prospective parliamentary candidates are taking place in Bradford West, Birmingham Sparkbrook/Small Heath, and Bethnal Green and Bow, all with very high concentrations of Asians, in the next few weeks. In addition to the three sitting MPs of Asian origin, it appears that, so far, two other Asian candidates have been given safe or winnable Labour seats. However, this situation could change once the selection for all the parliamentary seats has taken place. One thing is clear: the number of Asian-origin MPs after the next general election will certainly increase.

Looking at the representation of Asians in local councils, it appears that slow progress has been made. In 1974, in the London borough elections, only twelve Asian and other ethnic minority councillors were elected. Ten of them represented the Labour Party and two belonged to the Conservative Party. In 1978, the number of ethnic minority councillors reached thirty-five. They included twenty-nine Labour, five Conservatives and one independent, M. Gupta in the Northcote ward of Ealing, with the highest percentage of Asian population nationally. By 1982, this number had risen to seventy-nine in the London borough elections, in which a total number of 1,914 councillors were elected. Sixty-nine of these were elected for Labour, seven for the Conservatives, two for the Liberals and one as an independent. Out of the seventy-nine ethnic minority councillors, forty-two were Asians and thirty-seven Afro-Caribbeans. The number of elected ethnic minority councillors was only 4 per cent of the total in the thirty-two London boroughs, while the ethnic minority population at that time was estimated at about 15 per cent of the total population. The slow progress, however, continued and at the 1986 London borough elections, out of the 142 elected ethnic minority councillors, sixty-eight were of Asian origin, as shown in Table 11.4.

These results show that the representation of Asians and other ethnic minorities in London was still modest. At the local elections in 1990, further progress was made in London borough elections. Although their overall share was still 10 per cent, with 179 Asian and Afro-Caribbean councillors out of a total of 1,914, a significant number of thirty-seven additional councillors were elected.

Table 11.4 Asian councillors in London boroughs, 1986

Party	Asian	Afro-Caribbean	Other ethnic minority	Total
Labour	64	55	13	132
Conservative	2	4	1	7
Liberal/SDP	2	1	0	3
Total	68	60	14	142

Source: Author's survey 1986

The total number, however, did not reflect the 20 per cent ethnic minority population in London boroughs.

At the 1994 London boroughs elections, the number of Asian councillors increased to 139. This again shows progress, particularly in some boroughs, and Table 11.5 shows boroughs with five or more Asian councillors.

However, the situation outside London has been worse. In the 1973 local elections, only six ethnic minority councillors were elected, of whom one was Liberal and the rest all Labour. More recently, in some areas of high Asian concentration, slow progress, over time, has been made. In Birmingham, in 1982, out of the 375 local election candidates, twenty-three were from ethnic minority communities, but only five (Labour Party) candidates were elected. Four of them were Asians. After ten years, in 1992, the number of Asian councillors reached fourteen (with another four Afro-Caribbeans). They all belonged to the Labour Party and it was estimated that one fourth of Labour councillors in Birmingham belonged to ethnic minorities. By 1996 the number of Asian councillors in Birmingham

Table 11.5 London boroughs with five or more Asian councillors

Council	Total council	Asian
Brent	66	8
Ealing	71	15
Greenwich	62	7
Haringey	59	8
Hounslow	60	14
Lewisham	67	6
Newham	60	14
Redbridge	62	7
Tower Hamlets	50	14
Waltham Forest	57	10

Source: 1994 local elections

had reached sixteen, and again they all belonged to the Labour Party. Several of them are young Asians, and this applies to other areas as well. In Leicester, at the 1983 local elections, out of 173 candidates, thirty-three were from ethnic minorities, largely Asians. Eight of the nine Labour Party Asian candidates were elected, while no other ethnic minority candidate was elected because they were contesting unwinnable seats. In 1996, there were fourteen Asian councillors. Bradford council also had eleven Asian councillors, one of them representing the Conservative Party. For a long time, it had only three Asian councillors. Another council outside London with a significant number of Asian councillors, is Luton, which has eight Asian councillors, all Labour.

At county council level, it appeared in 1992 that there were twenty Asian councillors out of twenty-six ethnic minority councillors. They represented 0.93 per cent of all county councillors (2,849). Most of them were representing the Labour Party (Geddes 1993). In the ten counties monitored at the 1993 county council elections, twenty-seven out of the thirty-three Labour ethnic minority candidates (mostly Asians) were elected, but the eighteen Conservatives, four Liberal Democrats and five 'others' all lost (Le Lohe 1993). These included six Asian county councillors out of twenty-eight who were from the City of Leicester. The other county worth mentioning is Berkshire, where fourteen ethnic minority councillors were elected in 1993, mostly Asians. It was also reported that five Muslims were elected in Nottinghamshire at the 1993 county council elections. Most of them belonged to the Labour Party.

In the districts and metropolitan districts, the picture was fairly similar, i.e. most of the elected Asian councillors belonged to the Labour Party. Out of eighty-seven Asian district councillors, identified by a survey in 1992 (Geddes 1993), seventy-four belonged to the Labour Party, seven to the Conservative Party, three were Liberal Democrats and another three were identified as 'independents'. They were mostly Asian men (eighty-two) and only five were Asian women. In the metropolitan districts, a similar pattern emerged, with twenty-four Asian men representing the Labour Party compared with only one Asian woman councillor. Table 11.6 gives the details of Asian councillors compared with Afro-Caribbean councillors in 1992. The table also shows that Afro-Caribbean women were more likely to be involved in local politics than were Asian women.

Table 11.6 Asian and Afro-Caribbean councillors in England by gender, 1992

Ethnic group	Men	Women	Total
Asian	185	17	202
Afro-Caribbean	53	32	85
Total	238	49	287

Source: Geddes 1993

Overall, it appeared that, in 1996, the estimated number of Asian councillors had reached over 300 nationally, including Scotland, and most of them (88 per cent) belonged to the Labour Party. While a significant improvement has taken place in terms of Asian representation at local council level, we should not forget that these 300 councillors are out of almost 23,000 local councillors in England and Wales alone, and compared with the Asian population their number is very low. One further point is relevant here: while in local councils over 70 per cent of the ethnic minority councillors are of Asian origin, in the House of Commons only three out of the six ethnic minority origin MPs are Asians. To reflect the Asian population, there need to be twenty-five MPs of Asian origins. It is clear that all political parties and Asian communities need to do more at both national and local levels to achieve a fair representation. Young Asians, in particular, point out that they experience several obstacles to the selection of Asian candidates for 'safe' and 'winnable' seats. Some of them point out that racial discrimination is a contributory factor for Asian and other ethnic minority groups' under-representation in town halls and in the House of Commons.

The policies and actions taken by the political parties to encourage Asian participation in politics are important, as are the attitudes of their candidates towards such participation. We examine the results of three surveys of candidates in this context. Two were undertaken at the 1979 and 1983 general elections, and one at the 1990 local elections (for details see Anwar 1994). In both the 1979 and 1983 surveys, an overwhelming majority of candidates, (89 per cent and 94 per cent respectively) felt that ethnic minorities ought to be encouraged to take a more active role in British politics. The 1990 survey showed 97 per cent of respondents saying 'yes' to the question: 'Do you think people from ethnic minority groups should be encouraged to take a more active role in British politics?' When we asked what form their participation should take, in the 1979 survey, 77 per cent of candidates in the sample were in favour of ethnic minorities becoming more involved in the existing political structure. In the 1983 survey, 71 per cent mentioned that ethnic minorities should be encouraged to join and be active in political parties and the relevant organisations, and another 18 per cent responded in a general way, saying that they should take a full part in the democratic process. In 1990, we discovered that 87 per cent of the sample of candidates in local elections preferred the form of Asians and other ethnic minorities getting involved in the existing political parties. In all three surveys, there was an almost total rejection of the formation of a separate political party for ethnic minorities.

As part of the 1990 study, we also interviewed party agents. Like the party candidates, the political party representatives did not want Asians and other ethnic minorities to have separate political parties but wanted them to join the existing political structures. Both the Labour Party and Conservative Party representatives said that theirs was the best party to represent Asians' interests, and both parties claimed that they had the support of most of the Asians in their areas. However, Labour Party representatives were in a better position to give examples of Asian members, more Asian elected councillors and candidates than were other parties. They were also in a better position to give examples of their regular contacts with Asians. One respondent suggested the fear of rejection and/or discrimination as a possible problem limiting the involvement of Asians and other ethnic minorities.

In fact, more recently, several examples had been reported where many Asians, particularly young Asians, felt that they had been banned from becoming members of the Labour Party or problems had been created for Asians standing as candidates. For example, some Asian Labour Party activists had tried to increase the membership by recruiting more Asians, but some constituency parties had been suspended and inquiries had been set up to delay the selection process. Small Heath and Sparkbrook in Birmingham were such areas. Others included Bradford West, Nottingham East and Manchester Gorton. All these areas have a significant Asian presence. Several stories with sensational headlines had appeared in the press to highlight that Asians were trying to take over parliamentary constituency parties. Examples of headlines include: 'Muslims "bought" anti-Kaufman votes' (referring to Gerald Kaufman's parliamentary seat of Manchester Gorton: *The Times*, 4 October

1994); 'Entryism or racism: Labour turns down one in four Asians for party membership amid fears of a local take-over' (*Independent on Sunday*, 25 September 1994); 'Labour alarm at Asian take-over' (also in the *Independent on Sunday*); 'Asians seize on safest route to Westminster' (*The Times*, 30 September 1994); an editorial 'Labour's Asians, deselection, democracy and the New Labour Party' (also in *The Times*); and so on. The Manchester Gorton selection of the parliamentary constituency, in which an Asian, a Muslim and an ex-Labour councillor from Brent had challenged the sitting MP, in fact ended up with an inquiry by the Labour Party's NEC, and some Asians took the Labour Party to the High Court. Three Asians accused the Party of blocking the membership applications of 600 Asians in the Manchester Gorton constituency. There was also a BBC television programme on this selection, which concluded that without the intervention of the Labour Party and the Labour Party NEC, there was an equal chance of the Asian candidate, Mr Shahzad, winning the selection. However, it is worth adding here that there were several other examples of local wards and parliamentary constituencies where Asians felt that they were not being treated equally by the political parties, and some had even accused the parties of racial discrimination. In particular, many young Asians had expressed such views.

A complaint against the Labour Party was also made to the CRE, in which some Asian members in Birmingham accused the party of possible discrimination taking place in the membership and selection process. It was reported that, as a result, some discussions took place in 1996 between the legal director of the CRE and Labour Party officials. Second generation Asians are also in the forefront of the campaign to increase the representation of Asians at both national and local levels. A new group, the Association for Active Asians in Labour (AAAL), was formed in March 1995 to fight racial harassment and racial discrimination within the Labour Party. In October 1994, 211 Asians resigned from the Conservative Party, alleging that they had encountered racism there (*Muslim News*, 28 October 1994). More recently the Conservative Party has also been accused of barring Asians from the Hayes and Harlington Conservative Association (*News*, 2 November 1995), and the sitting MP, Terry Dicks, highlighted this problem by saying that the association's treatment of Asian people, who represent a stronghold of 10,000, was unfair. It appeared that a former party branch chair, Lynda Reed, was forced to resign after twenty years due to overt racism. She said, 'When I recommended a good local Conservative who happened to be Asian for the 1994 Council elections I was told it was out of the question and me and my Asian friends would not be welcome' (*News*, 2 November 1995). The Conservative Party chairman had been urged by Nirj Deva, the only Conservative Asian MP in Britain, to investigate the allegation. The Conservative Party was also recently accused of 'blatant racism in their selection of candidates' (*The Times*, 27 September 1995).

The Tower Hamlets Liberal Democrats were accused of distributing a leaflet in November 1993, as part of their campaign in the area, which was condemned by the Liberal Democrat leader as racist (*Daily Telegraph*, 11 November 1993). As a result of the report of an inquiry relating to this and another leaflet, it was recommended that three local Liberal Democrats be suspended from the party. There was also a feud about playing a 'race card' between the local Labour Party and the Liberal Democrats in Tower Hamlets (Anwar 1994).

It is clear from various reported stories of racial harassment and racial discrimination within the political parties, and from my interviews with Asian activists in all three political parties, that there are still some obstacles, such as procedures, practices and less favourable treatment of Asians and other ethnic minorities, to getting equality of opportunity within the political parties. Also, when 'race' is seen as an electoral advantage, it is used by political parties without due consideration to race relations. At the 1992 general election, all three major political parties included statements concerning migration and race relations in their party manifestos. They used different terminology and put different emphasis on various issues in this context. It was generally assumed that, in 1992, 'immigration' would not become an election issue. However, it was made an election issue by the Conservative Party towards the end of the election campaign when they felt that they were behind in opinion polls. It appears that this move won them some white votes, which perhaps made some difference in the outcome of a close election contest. The facts of immigration did not justify the rhetoric of the then Home Secretary and others in his party. The issue of immigration during the election campaign also revived the debate about the numbers and presence of ethnic minorities in Britain. It is worth adding here that, before the 1992 election, it was renewed by the speeches of Conservative MP Winston Churchill, who made non-white immigration an issue. All these debates no doubt helped the victory of the first BNP candidate in the Millwall by-election, where immigration and ethnic minorities were pre- sented as the main election issues. At the same time, these devel- opments contributed to an increasing number of racial attacks and racial harassment cases in the early 1990s, particularly in the East End of London. At the time of writing, there were discussions taking place about the proposed Immigration and Asylum Bill, which the Labour Party and the Liberal Democrats are likely to oppose. The signs are that, once again, the 'immigration card' could be played at the next general election in 1997. However, the main political parties need to be careful not to use the 'immigra- tion' or 'race card' in elections in ways that could benefit the BNP, or similar extreme right organisations: the BNP is proposing to put forward fifty candidates at the next general election. The main parties need to be more positive and vigilant to fight racism and anti-ethnic minority activities and propaganda.

All the political parties are failing to integrate Asians fully into the political process. On the other hand, in the long run there seems to be some hope, looking at the experience of Jews in Britain. They are a good example of integration in the political process. The estimated number of Jews in Britain is 300,000, but there are at present nineteen MPs of Jewish origin, and several Jews are mem- bers of the European Parliament (MEPs) and the House of Lords. It is a great achievement for a small community. Alderman (1983) has described in detail the struggle of Jews to get into the British Parliament. The highest number of Jewish MPs (forty-six) was elected in 1974. There have been several Jewish members of Cabi- net. At one time in Thatcher's government there were five cabinet members of Jewish origin. As far as voting patterns are concerned, recently more Jewish electors have been voting for the Conservative Party candidates than for the Labour and Liberal Democrat. Alderman (1993) discovered, in a survey in Finchley, that 63 per cent of ABC1 Jews had voted for the Conservative candidate and 18 per cent each for the Labour and Liberal Democrat candidates at the 1992 general election. Are Asians likely to follow such a path? It is clear from my detailed analysis that Asians are following the Jewish community not only in educational and occupational trends but also in other ways, such as home ownership, strong religious affiliation, and emphasis on the importance of family life. These values are more relevant, it is argued by the Conservative

Party, to the Conservative Party philosophy. Therefore, Asians are seen as 'natural Conservatives' and, in the long run, like the Jews, the majority are expected to join and to support the Conservative Party. The Conservative Central Office and leadership's efforts in this connection, mentioned above, are slowly being successful. However, it appears that due to their colour, their relatively recent arrival compared with the Jews', and some of the resistance shown by local Conservative associations, full integration of Asians into the political process in the near future will be delayed.

It must be pointed out that, on the whole, all three major political parties have failed to integrate Asians sufficiently, together with other ethnic minority groups, and young Asians are pointing this out regularly. The increased participation and representation of young Asians in the political process and the positive policies of political parties in this connection should help the integration of Asians in society.

In addition to the electoral involvement of young Asians, they also take political action through a large number of Asian and multi-ethnic organisations. In fact, the number of such organisations is very large and ethnic mobilisation takes place on a variety of issues at local, national and sometimes European levels. It is worth pointing out that some of the voluntary activities and political action have provided Asian young people with necessary contacts with the establishment and thus given them training for the formal political process. Some events have also made Asians more determined to mobilise. For example, the Rushdie affair has made Muslims in Britain more politicised and, as a consequence, they have been mobilised by community leaders on other issues as well. Many Muslims have actually realised that they are not being treated equally as a religious community. As a result, some young Muslims recently have become more ardent supporters of the genuine demands of the Muslims in Britain. Some young Muslims, in particular, point to non-representation of Muslims in the House of Commons and the House of Lords. This is seen as deliberate by some and anti-Muslim policy by others. I would like to add that the question of representation of Muslims at national level also has its symbolic value and we expect it to be rectified at the 1997 general election. On the whole, Asians generally, but young Asians in particular, are likely to have an increasing influence in British politics in the future as participants rather than as subjects of debate and controversy.

Chapter 12

Conclusions

It is demonstrated in this book that the presence of South Asian people in Britain has historical, colonial, political and economic perspectives. The Asian population in Britain has increased substantially since 1961, from just over 100,000 to an estimated 1.7 million in 1996. With this, the number of British-born and/or British-educated Asian young people has also increased. The younger age profile of Asians means that the number of young Asians is proportionately large, and is likely to increase in the future. It is estimated that the proportion of British-born Asians is now 53 per cent and will be over 60 per cent of the total Asian population by the year 2001. There are many more who entered Britain as small children and have in fact grown up in the country. Therefore, the demographic profile of Asians will be different as we enter the twenty-first century. They are British and can no longer be considered as 'immigrants', 'foreigners' or 'outsiders'. They are an integral part of Britain. *S. Asian origin pple*

We have noted in Chapter 2 that Asians are highly concentrated in some regions and local authority areas, compared with other areas. However, there are some differences, in terms of settlement, between the three Asian ethnic groups. The Indians are comparatively more wide-spread but relatively more concentrated in the south east and the Midlands regions. Bangladeshis are mainly concentrated in Greater London, while Pakistanis are comparatively less concentrated in the south east and found in greater numbers in the West Midlands, Yorkshire, the north west and Scotland. This pattern of settlement for Asian groups is the result of their migration process, as presented in Chapter 1, and it has implications for the educational and employment opportunities for young Asians. For example, because of the restructuring of industry in the 1980s

Indian benefit |social class/118?
P. B. both unemployed £k3dE?

and 1990s, in which a lot of manufacturing jobs disappeared, the 20 per cent of Pakistanis, compared with only 2 per cent of whites, who worked in the textile industry were disproportionately affected and, as a result, many of them became unemployed. In the south east, where more jobs were created during the same period in the service industry, the restructuring appears to have benefited Indians. However, many Bangladeshis who live close to the prosperous area of the City of London, where there are not many unskilled jobs, and who live in some of the poorest boroughs of London, have not benefited from this change. Bangladeshis and Pakistanis, both first generation and young people, had among the highest unemployment rates in Britain in 1993: Pakistanis 30 per cent and Bangladeshis 28 per cent compared with 15 per cent of Indians and less than 10 per cent of whites. The youth (16–24-year-old) unemployment rates in 1995–6 (Office for National Statistics 1996b) confirmed this trend. Over 30 per cent of Pakistani and Bangladeshi and over 20 per cent of Indian young persons were unemployed, compared with 12 per cent of their white peers. The very high unemployment rates and proportions of unskilled and manual jobs mean that many Pakistanis and Bangladeshis with large families have low incomes and are in poverty. This has implications for housing, health and the education of their children. The Fourth PSI Survey discovered that even Indians were well represented simultaneously amongst both the prosperous and the poor. For example, Indians were nearly twice as likely as whites to be financially in the top seventh of the self-employed, but, at the same time, twice as likely to be in the poorest fifth of non-pensioner households (Modood *et al.* 1997). No doubt an increasing rate of self-employment in the last twenty years has helped them to improve their incomes and also to avoid discrimination in the job market. However, the general trend among young Asians seems to be to aspire for professional jobs rather than work long and unsociable hours in catering and newsagent-type family-run small businesses, which, sometimes, are not even economical. For example, a recent survey found that a quarter of self-employed Asians worked more than sixty hours a week (Metcalf *et al.* 1996). The 1991 Census also showed social class differences between Indians, Pakistanis and Bangladeshis. Relatively more Indians (9.2 per cent) were in the professional category than Pakistanis (5.9 per cent) and Bangladeshis (4.9 per cent). Since we know that educational achievement is strongly linked to social class, we expect more Indian children to perform better.

It is clear that a greater number of Asian young people are staying on in education after the compulsory school-leaving age of 16. This is contributing to their A-level results and better qualifications. It is also done to overcome some of the disadvantage young Asians face at schools. However, there is a lot of family encouragement and support for young Asians to achieve higher qualifications and they seem to be responding. For example, Indians aged 18–29 had a higher percentage (15.2 per cent) of higher qualifications than whites (12.5 per cent). However, fewer Pakistanis (7.2 per cent) and Bangladeshis (3.4 per cent) in this age group had higher qualifications. This trend is also confirmed when we examine their participation in higher education. On the whole, it appears that, in the last twenty years, the educational achievement of all Asian young people has improved but the differences between Asian groups remain. For example, the Indian and African Asian young people are achieving better examination results, than Pakistani and Bangladeshi young people. However, there are area variations. Pakistanis in London, for example, are achieving better GCSE examination results than Pakistani pupils in Birmingham and Bradford (Anwar 1996).

The proportion of Asians in higher education is estimated to be almost 4 per cent of the total, which is a higher percentage than that of their numbers in the population. However, we should bear in mind that the Asian population is a young one and, combined with their higher educational aspirations, we should therefore expect more young Asians in education generally. The trend in the early 1990s shows that, despite the differential acceptance rate based on ethnicity compared with white applicants, the representation of Asians, particularly Indians and now also Pakistanis, in higher education is increasing and is likely to increase further in the future. It is worth pointing out that twenty years ago one in eight school leavers went into higher education, but now one in three do so.

It emerged from the analysis that the spread of subjects Asian young people choose to study in higher education is uneven. For example, more Asians apply for the subjects which require higher A-level points, such as medicine and law, compared with teacher training courses which require significantly lower A-level points (almost half of the medicine and law scores). The 1994–5 higher education figures showed that 12 per cent of Indian and 10 per cent of Pakistani/Bangladeshi students were studying medicine, compared with 7 per cent of whites. Six per cent of whites and only 3 per cent of Indians and 4 per cent of Pakistani/Bangladeshi students were in teacher training (Office for National Statistics 1996a). This pattern is found partly because many Asian parents put pressure on their children to go for medicine and law and partly because young Asians see medicine and law as well-respected professions with good incomes. It is also worth pointing out that many of these young Asians are sons and daughters of Asian doctors, who have a significant representation in the National Health Service. On the other hand, the representation of Asians as teachers and as academics in higher education institutions is very small. The same applies to some other professions and services, such as social work, the police and the probation service. It appeared from our analysis in Chapter 4 that 34 per cent of Asian young people did not receive any advice on leaving school. We also discovered that few Asian young people received advice from their parents and family, although the general view is that Asian young people do get such advice from their family and friends.

We can conclude from the evidence in Chapter 4 that Asian young people had unrealistic aspirations for some jobs. For example, 15 per cent claimed to have wanted professional jobs but only 3 per cent actually got such jobs after leaving full-time education. On the other hand, only 6 per cent of Asian young people said that they wanted an unskilled manual job but in fact 23 per cent of Asians had actually gone into such work. Therefore, there seems to be a need to make realistic careers advice available for Asian young people both in schools and in further and higher education institutions.

We found that the majority of Asian parents and young Asians were pessimistic about young people finding a job after completing full-time education. It was clear from the responses that racial discrimination was seen by many Asians as a contributory factor to the high unemployment among Asians. For example, the unemployment rate for 16–24-year-old Pakistanis and Bangladeshis, in 1991, was more than double that of white young people, and even for Indians it was significantly higher; this trend is confirmed by the recent figures referred to above. It is worth pointing out that the unemployment rate for young Asian females was also striking, particularly for Pakistanis and Bangladeshis. However, the supportive family structure has lessened the blow of unemployment for many young Asians.

We have also shown in Chapter 4 that higher qualifications do not generally help to remove racial differences in employment levels. Asian graduates appeared to experience greater difficulties than whites in obtaining employment. They had to make more applications than their white peers and they perceived more difficulties in gaining employment because of their ethnicity.

It is worth pointing out that, when the 1975 survey was undertaken, the unemployment rate for Asians was estimated at just over 6 per cent, compared with 5 per cent for the general population. However, in 1996, the unemployment situation of Asians, both first and second generation, compared with that for whites looks very bad. Our analysis shows that racial discrimination is a major contributory factor to these ethnic differences and this is perceived by both Asians and white people, very few saying that employers are not prejudiced. In early 1997 the Education and Employment Secretary, Gillian Shephard, admitted that many ethnic minority candidates faced discrimination when applying for jobs (speech in London, 28 January 1997). She also said that unemployment among ethnic minorities was twice as high as for white people.

We found too that those Asians who were in jobs were more likely to mention discrimination in terms of promotion, getting pay rises, being given the worst or hardest jobs, name calling and being generally treated badly because of their colour and ethnic group. We also found that 70 per cent of careers advisors and job centre workers felt that a few employers were racially prejudiced, and over 40 per cent of them said that they had received discriminatory instructions at least once in a twelve-month period. It is clear that most people, white and Asians, feel that employers discriminate on racial grounds, but some Asians also feel that employers discriminate because of their religion. The 1994 PSI Survey (Modood *et al.* 1997) found that 40 per cent of Asians felt that they had been discriminated against because of their religion, usually combined with their race. Therefore, it is clear that they face double discrimination, racial and religious. It appears that white people express more prejudice against Asians and Muslims than against Caribbeans. Recent examples include Muslim girls being refused jobs because of their dress and Sikh pupils refused school admission because of their turbans. Also, British Airways was recently accused of racial discrimination by two Sikh young people who were refused cabin stewards' jobs because of their turbans and beards.

In addition to racial and religious discrimination, many Asians are racially harassed and some have reported racial attacks, as analysed in Chapter 6. As a consequence, a significant number of Asians worry about being racially harassed and or attacked. More than a third of young Asians in our survey said they themselves or a family member or a friend had been attacked, mainly on a racial basis. This means that, overall, a substantial number of Asians are attacked because of their colour and/or culture; and racial harassment affects families, not just individuals. Very few victims of racial harassment complained to the police since, as we found, many believed that the police did not take any action. As a result, Asian young people were not very optimistic about police protection from racial harassment and therefore a majority of them believed in self-defence groups to protect themselves (Chapter 6). Such views have clear implications for their attitudes towards race relations.

In the last twenty years, the attitudes of Asians towards race relations have changed dramatically. In 1975, for example, 43 per cent of Asians felt that race relations were getting better, but, in 1983, only 19 per cent of young people felt that race relations were better and 16 per cent felt that they would get better over the next five years, while 29 per cent said race relations would get worse in the future. On the other hand, two-thirds of white people and 56 per cent of Asian people, in 1991, thought Britain was a very or fairly racist society (see Chapter 6). An ICM survey in 1995 also showed that two-thirds of the respondents admitted to being racist. The change in attitudes in the last twenty years shows that, on the one hand, more white people are prepared to accept that racism is a problem and, on the other hand, young Asians have become more aware of their rights as British citizens and have become vocal about the issues of inequality and different treatment because of their colour, culture and religion.

With regard to cultural issues, presented in Chapters 7–9, interesting developments within the Asian communities are taking place. For example, the prestige of the family was almost unanimously regarded as being sacrosanct. A significant number of Asian families still lived and or functioned as extended or joint families. These families were both horizontally and vertically extended. Most unmarried young Asians, but also many married young people, lived with their parents and, where they were unable to live together because of the difficulties of finding large enough houses, they lived separately but functioned as joint/extended families. Although some young Asians felt that they wanted more privacy, there was almost unanimous agreement that they had a duty to look after their parents, and generally these attitudes and this behaviour are likely to continue in the foreseeable future. Similarly, the practice of arranged marriages among Asians is likely to continue, but with a flexible approach. My research has shown that, in the 1990s, there was a lot of discussion and negotiation taking place between parents and young people, compared with the 1970s, before a decision about a partner was taken. This applied to both Asian boys and girls. However, there was a minority of young people, particularly African Asians, who made their own decisions about their marriage partners. In a minority of Asian families, the issue of arranged marriages sometimes leads to conflict between parents and young people, and some of these stories get disproportionate media coverage. It is worth stressing that, because of the resistance of young Asians, particularly Asian girls, fewer marriages are now arranged in the countries of origin and the trend is downward. There were also very few inter-ethnic unions (Berrington 1996). It is worth pointing out that the myth of return among first generation Asians, compared with the 1970s, has now diminished and, as a result, their attitudes and practices on various cultural aspects have become more flexible and sometimes changed. However, I have found that, while some of the forms are modified, the ceremonies which take place at Asian weddings in the subcontinent are being organised in Britain in a similar way. Similarly, transplantation of other religio-cultural norms is also taking place in the British context.

Religion is an important area for all Asian groups in ways which make them different from other ethnic groups. For an overwhelming majority of Asians, religion was the main basis for their ethnic identity. However, there were differences between Asian groups. For example, almost three-quarters of Muslims thought religion was very important for the way they lived their life, compared with less than half of Hindus and Sikhs saying this. Many parents worry that there is not enough done in schools to teach their religions and cultures. We found that 56 per cent of young white people never prayed, compared with only 18 per cent young Asians. The 1994 PSI Survey (Modood *et al.* 1997) also found similar trends for young Asians. However, while almost two-thirds of Muslims attended prayer meetings or went to a place of worship once a week or more, four out of ten Sikhs and only less than one in three Hindus did so. Such religious-group attitude differences are also found between Muslims, on the one hand, and Sikhs and Hindus, on the other, on issues like single-sex schooling, and establishing schools of one's own religion. For example, significantly few Hindu and Sikh young people supported single-sex schooling for their daughters compared with Pakistani and Bangladeshi young people. For all Asian groups, young people were less likely to prefer single-sex schooling than were older people, but the pattern regarding religious-group differences, as mentioned above, did not change significantly. Similarly, while, almost three out of ten Muslims would prefer a school of their own religion, less than one in ten Hindus and Sikhs expressed this view.

Differences between Muslims, and Sikhs and Hindus, also emerged on the question of freedom for girls. Relatively more Muslim parents, compared with Hindus and Sikh parents, agreed that they would not let their teenage daughters go to places where white girls go. Fewer young people were in favour of restricting the leisure activities of teenage girls but more young Muslims were in favour (see Chapter 9). For Asian girls, wearing Western dress is also seen as an indication of freedom. Opposition among parents to young Asian girls wearing Western clothes seemed to have declined between 1975 and 1983, although the differences between groups, with Muslims expressing more opposition than Hindus and Sikhs, remained. In fact, the significantly higher tendency of Muslim young women always to wear Asian clothes compared with very few Hindu and Sikh women was also discovered by the 1994 PSI Survey (Modood *et al.* 1997). *Religion some rty Muslim < Sikh Hindus*

More young Asians than their parents wanted to be with other Asians most of their spare time. Generally, the main differences in attitudes were linked to religion and social class. For example, working-class Asians, both parents and young people, wanted to spend their spare time with other Asians more than did middle-class Asians. Among religious groups, more young Muslims preferred to spend their spare time with other Asians than did Sikh and Hindu young people.

The generational differences also appeared in the preferences for living in a particular area. Seven out of ten parents, compared with less than half of young Asians, agreed that they enjoyed living in an area where there were lots of other Asian families. The reasons for these attitudes are presented in Chapter 9. However, it was clear that more young Asians would like to live outside such areas. It is not because they did not like the community facilities and other Asian families in such areas, but because these areas were run-down inner-city areas with low-quality housing. It is true that most of the Indians and Pakistanis were owner-occupiers but relatively fewer lived in detached or semi-detached properties, compared with whites, although there were differences between Asian groups, as presented in Chapter 5. While over 50 per cent of Indians lived in detached or semi-detached houses, only 28 per cent of Pakistanis and 20 per cent of Bangladeshis did so. It is worth stressing that, in the 1990s, a significant improvement for all Asian groups in this respect had taken place compared with the 1970s and 1980s. However, the ethnic differences remained on other housing condition indicators as well. For example, nationally about 30 per cent of Pakistani and over 47 per cent of Bangladeshi households were overcrowded, compared with 13 per cent of Indian and less than 2 per cent of white households in this situation (1991 Census). In Birmingham, we discovered that almost two-thirds of Pakistani and 56 per cent of Bangladeshi households were without central heating, compared with 30 per cent of Indian households.

From all the evidence in the book, we can conclude that Pakistanis and Bangladeshis are the most disadvantaged groups, compared with Indians and also compared with whites. Indians and African Asian young people are, comparatively, achieving better in education, have greater participation in higher education and, as a result, have better higher qualifications than Pakistani and Bangladeshi young people. The same pattern applies to the participation of young Indians in the economic field, compared with Pakistani and Bangladeshi young people. The unemployment rate among Indians is also lower, though higher than white people's, compared with very high unemployment among Pakistanis and Bangladeshis. These differences are partly due to their skills and qualifications but also to where these groups are located in terms of regions. For example, the majority of Pakistanis are living in regions with higher unemployment rates, and the unskilled jobs the majority of them were doing, before the restructuring of industry took place have now disappeared. However, it is worth mentioning that while, generally and also in the regions where Asians are, the unemployment rate among white people is coming down, for Pakistanis and Bangladeshis the unemployment rate is going up. This also applies to British-educated young Asians.

In politics, young Asians' participation has increased significantly as members and electors, but the political representation of Asians generally and Asian young people in particular has made only slow progress. In fact, young Asians feel frustrated that obstacles are in their way when they become members, seek office, or try to become party candidates. In politics, all the main political parties have failed to integrate Asians within their structures. However, many young Asians I have spoken to felt that political parties could not rely on Asian support without giving something in return. It appears that in the future young Asians will increasingly challenge the political parties on their under-representation and also on the relevance of their policies to a multi-racial and multi-cultural Britain.

Most policy makers we interviewed accepted that Asians and white young people faced different problems, and many said that Asians had different needs in education, careers advice and recreation and had different employment prospects. But little was done by policy makers to meet those different needs of young Asians. At the same time policy makers were obsessed with the cultural and language differences of Asians and saw them as the causes of most of the difficulties Asian young people faced in education, careers advice, training and the job market. In fact their views were almost the opposite to those of young Asians and Asian parents on these matters. Chairs and vice-chairs of relevant committees on the whole lacked full knowledge about the policies and procedures of their councils relevant to young Asians.

The professionals we interviewed also lacked a comprehensive knowledge about the problems of young Asians and they often saw them in terms of their own specialised areas. However, a few well-informed professionals saw Asian young people facing racial prejudice and discrimination but also having difficulties because of their cultural backgrounds.

Asian young people generally felt that they were not being treated equally and that they were in practice second-class citizens. They also felt that their parents have, on the whole, tolerated prejudice, discrimination and harassment, perhaps as the price of settling in Britain. However, it appears that young Asians were not prepared to accept racial discrimination and harassment, particularly when they were working hard to integrate in education, business and other fields. Compared with the 1970s, young Asians in the 1990s were asserting their Britishness, and were more articulate and more aggressive in their approach to highlighting unfair treatment by the institutions of society. One example of this was the troubles in Bradford in 1995 and the unrest in Birmingham and other areas in 1996, in which young Asians were involved (Chapter 6). Generally, authority was resented, the pleas of Asian leaders and parents were ignored, and demands were made to tackle racial discrimination and their unequal treatment by the structures of society. It is interesting that, generally, compared with the 1970s, more recently young Asians were less critical of Asian organisations' ineffectiveness in recognising and meeting the needs of young Asians. This was partly due not only to the improved communication between first and second generation Asians, but also because several young Asians were now involved in or were leading such organisations. Young Asians also feel that while Asian organisations play an important role in the religio-cultural sphere, they are unable to tackle racial disadvantage and racial discrimination, which the structures of society need to remove. It is clear from our evidence that some of the structural barriers are likely to continue for young Asians in the foreseeable future because of their skin colour and religious and cultural differences. These differences will be used by some as a basis for discrimination and hostility against them. For example, Islamophobia has recently become 'more explicit, more extreme and more dangerous' (*Independent*, 21 February 1997).

It appears that, compared with the 1970s, the attitudes of Asian parents regarding cultural issues have become more tolerant. As a result, there was an improvement in communication, more discussions and negotiations were taking place between parents and young Asians, and therefore the chances of generational conflict were minimised. On the whole, young Asians wanted to learn more about their culture and religion and felt that they needed more facilities and opportunities to learn these at school and in the communities. Generally, there was a significant religio-cultural conformity, although the differences between religious groups remained. For example, young Muslims seemed to be more 'conservative' in their outlook and had a higher conformity to religio-cultural norms than did Hindu and Sikh young people. These differences were partly religious and partly linked to social class, educational backgrounds, areas of origin and the time of migration to Britain. Overall, the approach of young Asians seems to be continuity and change, sometimes leading to tensions between generations. In brief, young Asians are adopting a new culture which is a synthesis of the 'old' and the 'new'.

Appendix
Surveys

The 1975 Survey: As part of this study 1,117 young Asians (13–21 years of age) living at home and 944 Asian parents who had children in that age range were interviewed from nine areas throughout the country in 1975. In addtion 175 'experts' were interviewed from twenty-four areas known to contain a significant number of Asians. An expert was defined as a person knowledgeable about the Asian community, either because of his or her position as a recognised community/religious leader or because of his or her professional relationship with the community. Forty young Asians who had left home as a result of differences of opinion with their parents were also interviewed. The fieldwork was carried out by the Opinion Research Centre for the Community Relations Commission under the supervision of the author.

The 1983/4 Survey: The Commission for Racial Equality commissioned the Harris Research Centre to undertake fieldwork for a major study of young people. The author had designed and supervised the study. The focus of the study was on education, employment and the transition between the two. Other areas covered were housing, relations with the police, leisure and race relations. An additional section on religio-cultural attitudes was included for Asian respondents in order to update the findings of the 1975 survey. Altogether 1,858 young people aged 15–24 were interviewed in areas of high ethnic minority concentration in Britain. The sample comprised 570 Asians, 507 Afro-Caribbeans, 427 whites, 122 Cypriots, 106 Chinese and 118 Arabs and other ethnic minorities.

In addition 509 parents who had children in the age range 15–24 were interviewed from the same areas. The parents' sample included 212 Asian, 147 Afro-Caribbean, 49 Cypriot and 101 white respondents. Interviews with young people and parents took place during 1983.

In 1984 interviews were carried out with professionals and local policy makers. Altogether 229 interviews were conducted, which included: eighty-five teachers, forty-eight careers advisors, fifty-two job centre workers and forty-four local councillors. This approach, like the 1975 survey, helped to relate the experiences of young Asians and others to their family, religious, cultural, social and political environment.

The Fourth Survey of Ethnic Minorities (1994): This is the fourth in a series of surveys of ethnic minorities in Britain undertaken first by the Political and Economic Planning (PEP) in 1966 and 1974; and then by the Policy Studies Institute (PSI) in 1982 and 1994. The 1994 survey was jointly undertaken by the PSI and the SCPR (Smith and Prior 1996; Modood *et al.* 1997). Interviews were completed with a nationally representative sample of 5,196 South Asians, Caribbeans and Chinese, and 2,867 whites. Out of the ethnic minority sample 3,777 interviews were with South Asians.

References

Alderman, G. (1983) *The Jewish Community in British Politics*, Oxford: Clarendon Press.

Alderman, G. (1993) 'The Jewish Dimension in British Politics since 1945', *New Community*, 20 (1).

Allen, S. (1971) *New Minorities, Old Conflicts: Asian and West Indian Migrants in Britain*, New York: Random House.

American Jewish Committee (1993) *British Survey*, London: American Jewish Committee.

Amin, K. and Richardson, R. (1992) *Politics For All*, London: Runnymede Trust.

Anwar, M. (1973) 'Pakistani Participation in the 1972 Rochdale By-Election', *New Community*, 2 (4).

Anwar, M. (1974) 'Pakistani Participation in the 1973 Local Elections', *New Community*, 3 (1–2).

Anwar, M. (1975) 'Asian Participation in the 1974 Autumn Election', *New Community*, 4 (3).

Anwar, M. (1976) *Between Two Cultures*, London: Community Relations Commission.

Anwar, M. (1979) *The Myth of Return*, London: Heinemann.

Anwar, M. (1980) *Votes and Policies*, London: CRE.

Anwar, M. (1981) *Race Relations in 1981*, London: CRE.

Anwar, M. (1982) *Young People and the Job Market*, London: CRE.

Anwar, M. (1984) *Ethnic Minorities and the 1983 General Election*, London: CRE.

Anwar, M. (1985) *Pakistanis in Britain*, London: New Century Publications.

Anwar, M. (1986) *Race and Politics*, London: Tavistock.

Anwar, M. (1990) 'Ethnic Classification, Ethnic Monitoring and the 1991 Census', *New Community*, 16 (4).

Anwar, M. (1991a) 'Ethnic Minorities' Representation: Voting and Electoral Politics in Britain, and the Role of Leaders', in Werbner, P. and Anwar, M. (eds), *Black and Ethnic Leaderships*, London: Routledge.

Anwar, M. (1991b) *Race Relations Policies in Britain: Agenda for the 1990s*, Coventry: Centre for Research in Ethnic Relations.

Anwar, M. (1993) *Muslims in Britain: 1991 Census and Other Statistical Sources*, Birmingham: Centre for the Study of Islam and Christian–Muslim Relations.

Anwar, M. (1994) *Race and Elections*, Coventry: Centre for Research in Ethnic Relations.

Anwar, M. (1995) 'New Commonwealth Migration to the UK', in Cohen, R. (ed.), *Cambridge Survey of World Migration*, Cambridge: Cambridge University Press.

Anwar, M. (1996) *British Pakistanis*, Birmingham: Pakistan Forum/Birmingham City Council.

Anwar, M. and Ali, A. (1987) *Overseas Doctors: Experience and Expectations*, London: CRE.

Anwar, M. and Kohler, D. (1975) *Participation of Ethnic Minorities in the General Election, October 1974*, London: Community Relations Commission.

Ashby, B., Morrison, A. and Butcher, A. (1970) 'The Abilities and Attainment of Immigrant Children', *Research in Education*, 4.

Aurora, G. S. (1967) *The New Frontiersmen: A Sociological Study of Indian Immigrants in the United Kingdom*, Bombay: Popular Parakashan.

Ballard, R. (ed.) (1994) *Desh Pardesh: The South Asian Presence in Britain*, London: Hurst.

Ballard, R. (1996) 'The Pakistanis: Stability and Introspection', in Peach, C. (ed.), *Ethnicity in the 1991 Census*, vol. 2, London: OPCS.

Berrington, A.-C. (1996) 'Marriage Patterns and Inter-Ethnic Unions', in Coleman, D. and Salt, J. (eds), *Ethnicity in the 1991 Census*, vol.1, London: OPCS.

Bhachu, P. (1986) *The Twice Migrants*, London: Tavistock.

Birmingham City Council (1995 and 1996) *GCSE Results by Ethnic Groups*, Birmingham: Department of Education.

Boodhoo, M.-J. and Baksh, A. (1981) *The Impact of Brain Drain on Development: A Case Study of Guyana*, Georgetown: University of Guyana.

Brah, A. (1978) 'South Asian Teenagers in Southall, Their Perceptions of Marriage, Family and Ethnic Identity', *New Community*, 6 (3).

Brah, A. and Shaw, S. (1992) *Working Choices: South Asian Young Muslim Women and the Labour Market*, Research Paper No. 91, London: Department of Employment.

Breeze, E., Trevor, G. and Wilmot, A. (1991) *General Household Survey*, London: OPCS/HMSO.

Brennan, J. and McGeevor, P.C. (1990) *Ethnic Minorities and the Graduate Labour Market*, London: CRE.

Bristow, M. (1976) 'Britain's Response to the Ugandan Asian Crisis', *New Community*, 5(3).

Brown, C. (1984) *Black and White Britain*, London: Policy Studies Institute.

Brown, C. and Gay, P. (1985) *Racial Discrimination: 17 Years After the Act*, London: PSI.

Cabinet Papers (1950) 'Coloured People from British Colonial Territories', (50) 113, Public Records Office.

Cabinet Papers (1956) 'Colonial Immigrants', Report of the Committee of Ministers, Public Records Office.

Cavanagh, T. E. (1984) *The Impact of the Black Electorate*, Washington, DC: Joint Centre for Political Studies.

Clough, E. and Drew, D. with Wojciechowski, T. (1985) *Futures in Black and White: Two Studies of the Experiences of Young People in Sheffield and Bradford*, Sheffield: Pavic Publications and Sheffield City Polytechnic.

Commission for Racial Equality (1984a) *Race and Council Housing in Hackney*, London: CRE.

Commission for Racial Equality (1984b) *Race and Housing in Liverpool: A Research Report*, London: CRE.

Commission for Racial Equality (1985a) *Immigration Control Procedures*, London: CRE.

Commission for Racial Equality (1985b) *Annual Report*, London: CRE.

Commission for Racial Equality (1985c) *Race and Mortgage Lending*, London: CRE.

Commission for Racial Equality (1987a) *Chartered Accountancy: Training Contracts*, London: CRE.

Commission for Racial Equality (1987b) *Living in Terror: A Report on Racial Violence and Harassment in Housing*, London: CRE.

Commission for Racial Equality (1988) *Investigation into St George's Hospital Medical School*, London: CRE.

Commission for Racial Equality (1989a) *Mandatory Visas*: London: CRE.

Commission for Racial Equality (1989b) *Racial Discrimination in Liverpool City Council*, London: CRE.

Commission for Racial Equality (1989c) *Housing Policies in Tower Hamlets: An Investigation*, London: CRE.

Commission for Racial Equality (1990) *Sorry It's Gone; Testing for Racial Discrimination in the Private Rented Housing Sector*, London: CRE.

Commission for Racial Equality (1993) *Evidence to the Select Committee of the House of Commons on Racial Attacks and Harassment*, London: CRE.

Community Relations Commission (1977) *Urban Deprivation, Racial Inequality and Social Policy*, London: CRC.

Cosgrave, P. (1990) *The Lives of Enoch Powell*, London: Pan.

Craft, M. and Craft, A. (1982) *The Participation of Ethnic Minorities in Further and Higher Education*, London: Nuffield Foundation.

Deakin, N. (ed.) (1965) *Colour and the British Electorate*, London: Pall Mall Press.

Deakin, N. (1970) *Colour, Citizenship and British Society*, London: Panther.

Department of Employment (1991) *Labour Force Surveys 1987–89*, London: HMSO.

Department of Employment (1993) *Labour Force Survey*, London: HMSO.

Department of Environment (1994) *Index of Local Conditions*, London: DOE.

Desai, R. (1963) *Indian Immigrants in Britain*, London: Oxford University Press.

Dhaya, B. (1974) 'The Nature of Pakistani Ethnicity in Industrial Cities in Britain', in Cohen, A. (ed.), *Urban Ethnicity*, London: Tavistock.

Dines, M. (1973) 'Ugandan Asians One Year Later: Cool Reception', *New Community*, 2 (4).

Drew, D. and Gray, J. (1990) 'The Fifth Year Examination Results of Black Young People in England and Wales', *Educational Research*, 32 (3).

Drew, D. and Gray, J. (1991) 'The Black–White Gap in Examination Results: A Statistical Critique of a Decade's Research', *New Community*, 17 (2).

Drew, D., Gray, J. and Sime, N. (1992) *Against the Odds: The Education and the Labour Market Experiences of Black Young People*, Sheffield: Employment Department.

Driver, G. (1980) *Beyond Under-Achievement*, London: CRE.

Driver, G. and Ballard, R. (1979) 'Comparing Performance in Multi-Cultural Schools – South Asian Students at 16 Plus', *New Community*, 7 (2).

Drury, B. (1991) 'Sikh Girls and the Maintenance of an Ethnic Culture', *New Community*, 17 (3).

Eggleston, S.J., Dunn, D. K. and Anjali, M. (1986) *Education for Some: The Educational and Vocational Experience of 15–18-Year-Old Members of Minority Ethnic Groups*, Stoke on Trent: Trentham Books.

Engels, F. (1952) *The Conditions of the Working Class in England in 1844*, London: George Allen & Unwin.

Esmail, A. Nelson, P., Primorolo, D. and Toma, T. (1995) 'Acceptance into Medical Schools and Racial Discrimination', *British Medical Journal*, 310.

Essen, J. and Ghodsian, M. (1979) 'The Children of Immigrants: School Performance', *New Community*, 7 (3).

Evans, P. (1971) *The Attitudes of Young Immigrants*, London: Runnymede Trust.

Foot, P.C. (1965) *Immigration and Race in British Politics*, Harmondsworth: Penguin.

Fryer, P. (1984), *Staying Power: The History of Black People in Britain*, London: Pluto Press.

Geddes, A. (1993) 'Asian and Afro-Caribbean Representation in Elected Local Government in England and Wales', *New Community*, 20 (1).

Ghuman, P.A.S. (1975) *The Cultural Context of Thinking: A Comparative Study of Punjabi and English Boys*, Slough: NFER.

Ghuman, P.A.S. (1994) *Coping With Two Cultures*, Clevedon: Multilingual Matters.

Gillborn, D. and Gipps, C. (1996) *Recent Research on the Achievements of Ethnic Minority Pupils*, London: Office for Standards in Education.

Gordon, P. (1990) *Racial Violence and Harassment*, London: Runnymede Trust.

Hartley-Brewer, M. (1965) 'Smethwick', in Deakin, N. (ed.), *Colour and the British Electorate 1964*, London: Pall Mall Press.

Haynes, J. (1971) *Educational Assessment of Immigrant Pupils*, Slough: NFER.

Health Education Authority (1994) *Black and Minority Ethnic Groups in England*, London: HEA.

Heineman, B. (1972) *The Politics of the Powerless: A Study of the Campaign Against Racial Discrimination*, London: Oxford University Press.

Hibberd, M. and Shapland, J. (1993) *Violent Crime in Small Shops*, London: Police Foundation.

Higher Education Statistics Agency (1995) *Ethnicity in Higher Education*, Cheltenham: HESA.

HMSO (1949) *The Royal Commission on Population Report*, Cmnd 7695, London: HMSO.

Home Affairs Committee (1986) *Racial Attacks and Harassment*, London: HMSO.

Home Affairs Committee (1989 and 1994) *Racial Attacks and Harassment*, London: HMSO.

Home Office (1963–7) *Commonwealth Immigrant Act 1962: Control of Immigration Statistics*, London: HMSO.

Home Office (1981) *Racial Attacks: Report of a Home Office Study*, London: HMSO.

Home Office (1984) *Control of Immigration Statistics: United Kingdom*, London: HMSO.

Home Office (1989) *The Response to Racial Attacks and Harassment: Guidance for the Statutory Agencies*, Report of the Inter-Departmental Racial Attacks Group, London: Home Office.

Home Office (1992) *British Crime Survey*, London: HMSO.

Home Office (1993) *Evidence to the Select Committee of the House of Commons on Racial Attacks and Harassment*, London: HMSO.

Home Office (1993–6) *Control of Immigration Statistics*, London: Research and Statistics Department.

Hubbuck, J. and Carter, S. (1980) *Half a Chance?*, London: CRE.

Jackson, J.A. (1963) *The Irish in Britain*, London: Routledge & Kegan Paul.

Jeffers, S. (1991) 'Black Sections in the Labour Party: The End of Ethnicity and "Godfather" Politics', in Werbner, P. and Anwar, M. (eds), *Black and Ethnic Leaderships*, London: Routledge.

Jones, T. (1993) *Britain's Ethnic Minorities*, London: Policy Studies Institute.

Jowell, R., Witherspoon, S. and Brook, L. (1984) *British Social Attitudes*, Aldershot: Gower/SCPR.

Jowell, R., Witherspoon, S. and Brook, L. (1992) *British Social Attitudes*, Dartmouth: Dartmouth Publishing.

Karn, V., Kemeny, J. and Williams, P. (1985) *Home Ownership in the Inner City: Salvation or Despair*, Aldershot: Gower.

Keysel, F. (1988) 'Ethnic Background and Examination Results', *Educational Research*, 30 (2).

Kohler, D. (1973) 'Public Opinion and the Ugandan Asians', *New Community*, 2 (2).

Kohler, D. (1976) *Some of My Best Friends*, London: CRC.

Kondapi, C. (1951) *Indians Overseas 1938–49*, New Delhi: Oxford University Press.

Layton-Henry, Z. (1992) *The Politics of Immigration*, Oxford: Blackwell.

Le Lohe, M.J. (1975) 'Participation in Elections by Asians in Bradford', in Crewe, I. (ed.), *The Politics of Race*, London: Croom Helm.

Le Lohe, M.J. (1984) *Ethnic Minority Participation in Local Elections*, Bradford: University of Bradford.

Le Lohe, M.J. (1993) 'Political Issues', *New Community*, 20 (1).

Lingayah, S. (1987) *Mauritian Immigrants in Britain*, London: Mauritius Welfare Association.

London Borough of Ealing (1988) *Ealing's Dilemma: Implementing Race Equality in Education*, London: Ealing LA.

London Borough of Waltham Forest (1996) 'Analysis of GCSE Examination Results', Education Department.

MacDonald, J. and MacDonald, L.D. (1962) 'Chain Migration, Ethnic Neighbourhood Formation and Social Network', *Social Research*, 29 (4).

Maughan, B. and Rutter, M. (1986) 'Black Pupils' Progress in Secondary Schools II: Examination Achievements', *British Journal of Developmental Psychology*, 4 (1).

Mayhew, P., Elliot, D. and Dawd, S. (1989) *The 1988 British Crime Survey*, London: HMSO.

McIntosh, N. and Smith, D. (1974) *The Extent of Racial Discrimination*, London: PEP.

Metcalf, H., Modood, T. and Virdee, S. (1996) *Asian Self-Employment*, London: PSI.

Mirrless-Black, C. and Maung, N.A. (1994) *Racially Motivated Crime: A British Crime Survey Analysis*, Paper 82, London: Home Office Research and Statistics Department.

Modood, T. (1993) 'The Number of Ethnic Minority Students in British Higher Education: Some Grounds for Optimism', *Oxford Review of Education*, 19 (2).

Modood, T. and Shiner, M. (1994) *Ethnic Minorities and Higher Education: Why Are There Differential Rates of Entry?*, London: PSI.

Modood, T., Beishon, S. and Virdee, S. (1994) *Changing Ethnic Identities*, London: PSI.

Modood, T. and Berthoud, R., Lakey, J., Nazroo, J., Smith, P., Virdee, S. and Beishon, S. (1997) *Ethnic Minorities in Britain: Diversity and Disadvantage: The Fourth National Survey of Ethnic Minorities*, London: PSI.

Murphy, M. (1996) 'Household and Family Structure Among Ethnic Minority Groups', in Coleman, D. and Salt, J. (eds), *Ethnicity in the 1991 Census*, vol. 1, London: OPCS.

Nuttall, D. L., Goldstein, H., Prosser, R. and Rasbash, J. (1989) 'Differential School Effectiveness', *International Journal of Educational Research*, 13.

Office for National Statistics (1996a) *Social Focus on Ethnic Minorities*, London: HMSO.

Office for National Statistics (1996b) *Labour Force Surveys*, London: HMSO.

Office of Population Censuses and Surveys (1983) *Census 1981: National Report, Great Britain*, London: HMSO.

Office of Population Censuses and Surveys (1993) *1991 Census: Ethnic Group and Country of Birth (Great Britain)*, London: HMSO.

Office of Population Censuses and Surveys Immigrant Statistics Unit (1975) 'Country of Birth and Colour', *Population Trends*, 2.

Owen, D. (1993) *Ethnic Minorities in Britain: Age and Gender Structure*, NEMDA 1991 Census Statistical Paper No. 2, Coventry: Centre for Research in Ethnic Relations.

Owen, D. (1994) *South Asian People in Great Britain: Social and Economic Circumstances*, Coventry: NEMDA/Centre for Research in Ethnic Relations.

Owen, D. (1995) 'Trends in Unemployment Rates by Ethnic Groups since 1992', NEMDA Information Paper 95/1.

Parekh, B. (1983) 'Educational Opportunity in Multi-Ethnic Britain', in Glazer, N. and Young, K. (eds), *Ethnic Pluralism and Public Policy*, London: Heinemann.

PEP (Political and Economic Planning) (1948) *Population Policy in Great Britain*, London: PEP.

Petersen, W. (1958) 'A General Typology of Migration', *American Sociological Review*, 23.

Ranger, C. (1988) *Survey of Teachers*, London: CRE.

Rex, J. and Moore, R. (1967) *Race, Community and Conflict: A Study of Sparkbrook*, London: Oxford University Press for IRR.

Rex, J. and Tomlinson, S. (1979) *Colonial Immigrants in a British City*, London: Routledge & Kegan Paul.

Rose, E.J.B. with Deakin, N., Abrams, M., Jackson, V., Peston, M., Vanags, A.H., Cohen, B., Gaitskell, J. and Ward, P. (1969) *Colour and Citizenship*, London: Oxford University Press for IRR.

Royal Commission on Population (1949) *Report of the Royal Commission on Population*, Cmnd 7695, London: HMSO.

Rudat, K. (1994) *Health and Lifestyles: Black and Minority Ethnic Groups in England*, London: Health Education Authority.

Ruddock, J. (1994) *Racial Attacks: The Rising Tide*, London: Labour Party.

Scarman, Lord (1981) *The Brixton Disorders, 10–12 April 1981*, Cmnd 8427, London: HMSO.

Shukra, K. (1990) 'Black Sections in the Labour Party', in Goulbourne, H. (ed.), *Black Politics in Britain*, Aldershot: Avebury.

Simpson, A. and Stevenson, J.C. (1994) *Half a Chance, Still? Jobs, Discrimination and Young People in Nottingham*, Nottingham and District Racial Equality Council.

Skellington, R. (1996) *'Race' in Britain Today*, London: Sage.

Smith, D. (1976) *The Facts of Racial Disadvantage*, London: PEP.

Smith, D. and Tomlinson, S. (1989) *The School Effect: A Study of Multi-Racial Schools*, London: Policy Studies Institute.

Smith, P. and Prior, G. (1996) *The Fourth National Survey of Ethnic Minorities: Technical Report*, London: Social and Community Planning Research.

Smith, S. (1993) *Electoral Registration in 1991*, London: OPCS (Social Surveys Division).

Stopes-Roe, M. and Cochrane, R. (1990) *Citizens of this Country: The Asian-British*, Clevedon: Multilingual Matters.

Swann, Lord (1985) *Education For All*, London: HMSO.

Tanna, K. (1990) 'Excellence, Equality and Educational Reform: The Myth of South Asian Achievement Level', *New Community*, 16 (3).

Taylor, M. with Hegarty, S. (1985) *The Best of Both Worlds... ? A Review of Research into the Education of Pupils of South Asian Origin*, Windsor: NFER-Nelson.

Taylor, P. (1992) 'Ethnic Group Data for University Entry', Unpublished Research Report for the Committee of Vice-Chancellors and Principals, Coventry: Centre for Research in Ethnic Relations.

Taylor, P. H. (1976) *The Half-Way Generation*, Windsor: NFER.

Taylor, S. (1982) *The National Front in English Politics*, London: Macmillan.

Todd, J. and Butcher, B. (1982) *Electoral Registration in 1981*, London: OPCS.

UCCA (Universities' Central Council on Admissions) (1992) *Statistical Supplement to the Twenty-Ninth Report 1990–91*, Cheltenham: UCCA.

UCCA (Universities' Central Council on Admission) (1993) *Statistical Supplement to the Thirtieth Report 1991–92*, Cheltenham: UCCA.

Vatuk, S. (1972) *Kinship and Urbanisation*, Berkeley, CA: University of California Press.

Vertovec, S. (1994) 'Caught in an Ethnic Quandary: Indo-Caribbean Hindus in London', in Ballard, R. (ed.), *Desh Pardesh: The South Asian Presence in Britain*, London: Hurst.

Virdee, S. (1995) *Racial Violence and Harassment*, London: Policy Studies Institute.

Visram, R. C. (1986) *Ayahs, Lascars and Princes*, London: Pluto Press.

Walker, M. (1977) *The National Front*, London: Fontana.

Ward, R. (1973) 'What Futures for the Ugandan Asians?', *New Community*, 2 (4).

Warrier, S. (1994) 'Gujarati Prajapatis in London: Family Roles and Sociability Networks', in Ballard R. (ed.), *Desh Pardesh: The South Asian Presence in Britain*, London: Hurst.

Werbner, P. (1990) *The Migration Process*, Oxford: Berg.

Index